MXene-Based Emerging 2D Materials for Biomedical Applications

This book provides a well-focused and comprehensive overview of the history and background of MXene-based materials and their structure, synthesis, properties, and modifications for making various advanced materials. It covers in-depth processing parameters for making MXene-based materials for high-end applications, especially in the biomedical and pharmaceutical fields.

MXene-Based Emerging 2D Materials for Biomedical Applications examines the use of MXenes in the healthcare sector as therapeutic agents in pharmaceuticals and medicine. The book examines MXene use in diagnosis and analysis as biosensors, disease detection, gene and drug delivery, cancer therapy, bioimaging, and graphene oxide (GO)-based antibacterial materials. It also discusses its potential as a promising antioxidant and GO-based scaffold for cell culture. It provides a comprehensive introduction of advanced MXene-based materials for the biomedical field/health sector through an interdisciplinary approach of research in science and biomedical engineering. The authors indicate possible areas wherein the advanced MXene-based emerging materials can benefit combining diagnostics and therapeutic possibilities and multiplex systems, and highlights the unique and novel approach to developing advanced medical applications platforms and state-of-the-art directions for future research.

This book will guide bioengineering and material science students, scientists, and researchers to plan future research in this valuable field. It is a unique book that gives broad knowledge about MXene-based advanced materials under a single umbrella and demonstrates the usefulness of MXenes in the healthcare sector in multiple ways.

MXene-Based Emerging 2D Materials for Biomedical Applications

Edited By
Sarika Verma

CRC Press
Taylor & Francis Group
Boca Raton London New York

CRC Press is an imprint of the
Taylor & Francis Group, an **informa** business

Designed cover image: Shutterstock

First edition published 2025
by CRC Press
2385 NW Executive Center Drive, Suite 320, Boca Raton FL 33431

and by CRC Press
4 Park Square, Milton Park, Abingdon, Oxon, OX14 4RN

CRC Press is an imprint of Taylor & Francis Group, LLC

ISBN: 978-1-032-40304-5 (hbk)
ISBN: 978-1-032-40482-0 (pbk)
ISBN: 978-1-003-35328-7 (ebk)

DOI: 10.1201/9781003353287

Typeset in Palatino
by Newgen Publishing UK

Contents

About the Author vii

Contributors ix

1 **Exploring the Potential of MXene-Based 2D Materials in the Realm of Biomedical Advancements** **1**
Kamna Chaturvedi and Sarika Verma

2 **MXene-Based 2D Materials for Biosensing** **18**
M. Chandrashekhar Nayak and Kajal Yadav

3 **MXene-Based Emerging 2D Materials for Biomarkers (Electrodes)** **31**
Lizaranee Tripathy, Ashish K. Sarangi, Rajiv Lochan Bal, Puneet K. Singh, Snehasish Mishra, Ajit Behera, and Ranjan K. Mohapatra

4 **MXene-Based Emerging 2D Materials for Biomedical Photothermal and Photodynamic Therapeutic Applications** **50**
Kajal Yadav, Kamna Chaturvedi, Anju Singhwane, and Sarika Verma

5 **Significance of MXene in Tissue Engineering: A Review** **70**
Manal M. Khan, Gaurav Chaturvedi, Ved Prakash Rao, and Madhuri Arora

6 **MXene Marvels: Exploring the Insights and Applications of MXENE-Based Materials in Wearable Technology for Healthcare Systems** **86**
Kamna Chaturvedi, Neelam Kumari, Umesh Dwivedi, and Sarika Verma

7 **Emerging 2D Titanium Carbide MXene in Tissue Regeneration for Healthcare Applications** **108**
Anju Singhwane, Manal Khan, Ranjan Mohapatra, Avanish Kumar Sriastava, and Sarika Verma

8 **MXene-Based 'Therapeutic Agents'** **121**
Gagan Kant Tripathi, Shikha Katre, Pradeep Khiriya, Priyavand Bundela, Purnima Swarup Khare, and Priyanka Dixit

9 MXene-Based Materials for Wound Healing **137**
Manal M. Khan, Gaurav Chaturvedi, Ved Prakash Rao, and Madhuri Arora

Index 155

About the Author

Sarika Verma is currently working as Senior Principal Scientist and IP Coordinator at CSIR-Advanced Materials and Processes Research Institute (AMPRI), Bhopal, India. She has more than 16 years of experience in Research and Teaching in CSIR and CSIR-AMPRI, Bhopal Govt. of India, and other organizations. She was awarded a PhD in chemical sciences from Barakatullah University, India. She has 25 patents filed and has been intensively engaged in multiple R&D projects to design and develop advanced materials useful for different broad application spectrums such as cement free materials, radiation-shielding materials, polymeric composites, and biomedical and energy materials via novel techniques, such as 3D printing. She also has experience in transferring the know-how technology to industries like m/s Permalli Wallace, Apte Medical Systems, Pune.

Contributors

Arora, Madhuri
All India Institute of Medical Sciences, Bhopal 462026, India
Bhopal, Madhya Pradesh, India

Bal, Rajiv Lochan
Department of Mining Engineering, Orissa School of Mining Engineering, Keonjhar 758001, Odisha, India

Behera, Ajit
Department of Metallurgical & Materials Engineering, National Institute of Technology, Rourkela-769008, Odisha, India

Bundela, Priyavand
School of Nanotechnology, Rajiv Gandhi Proudyogiki Vishwavidyalaya (RGPV), Bhopal, M.P., India

Chaturvedi, Gaurav
All India Institute of Medical Sciences, Bhopal 462026, Madhya Pradesh, India

Chaturvedi, Kamna
Academy of Council Scientific and Industrial Research – Advanced Materials and Processes Research Institute (AMPRI), Bhopal (M.P.), 462026, India and Council of Scientific and Industrial Research – Advanced Materials and Processes Research Institute, Bhopal (M.P.), 462026, India

Dixit, Priyanka
Computer Science & Engg, University Institute of Technology, RGPV, Bhopal, M.P., India

Dwivedi, Umesh
Amity University Rajasthan, Jaipur, India

Gagan Kant Tripathi
School of Nanotechnology (SONT)
Rajiv Gandhi Proudyogiki Vishwavidyalaya (RGPV)
Bhopal (M.P.), India

Katre, Shikha
School of Nanotechnology, Rajiv Gandhi Proudyogiki Vishwavidyalaya (RGPV), Bhopal, M.P., India

Khan, Manal M.
All India Institute of Medical Sciences, Bhopal 462026, India

Khare, Purnima Swarup
School of Nanotechnology, Rajiv Gandhi Proudyogiki Vishwavidyalaya (RGPV), Bhopal, M.P., India

Khiriya, Pradeep
School of Nanotechnology, Rajiv Gandhi Proudyogiki Vishwavidyalaya (RGPV), Bhopal, M.P., India

Kumari, Neelam
Amity University Rajasthan, Jaipur, India

Mishra, Snehasish
School of Biotechnology, KIIT Deemed University, Bhubaneswar – 751024, Odisha, India

Mohapatra, Ranjan K.
Department of Chemistry, Government College of Engineering, Keonjhar – 758002, Odisha, India

Nayak, M. Chandrashekhar
Academy of Council Scientific and Industrial Research – Advanced Materials and Processes Research Institute (AMPRI), Bhopal (M.P.), 462026, India and Council of Scientific and Industrial Research – Advanced Materials and Processes Research Institute, Bhopal (M.P.), 462026, India

Rao, Ved Prakash
All India Institute of Medical Sciences, Bhopal 462026, India

Sarangi, Ashish K.
Department of Chemistry, Centurion University of Technology and Management, Balangir, Odisha, India

Singh, Puneet K.
School of Biotechnology, KIIT Deemed University, Bhubaneswar – 751024, Odisha, India

Singhwane, Anju
Council of Scientific and Industrial Research – Advanced Materials and Processes Research Institute, Bhopal (M.P.), 462026, India

Sriastava, Avanish Kumar
Council of Scientific and Industrial Research – Advanced Materials and Processes Research Institute, Bhopal (M.P.), 462026, India

Tripathy, Lizaranee
Department of Chemistry, Centurion University of Technology and Management, Balangir, Odisha, India

Venu, Divya
Council of Scientific and Industrial Research- Advanced Materials and Processes Research Institute, Bhopal (M.P.), 462026, India

Verma, Sarika
Academy of Council Scientific and Industrial Research – Advanced Materials and Processes Research Institute (AMPRI), Bhopal (M.P.), 462026, India and Council of Scientific and Industrial Research- Advanced Materials and Processes Research Institute, Bhopal (M.P.), 462026, India

Yadav, Kajal
Council of Scientific and Industrial Research- Advanced Materials and Processes Research Institute, Bhopal (M.P.), 462026, India

1

Exploring the Potential of MXene-Based 2D Materials in the Realm of Biomedical Advancements

Kamna Chaturvedi and Sarika Verma

1.1 Introduction

Over the past few years, the discipline of material science has witnessed a significant increase in the interest in 2D materials and their potential applications in a variety of domains encompassing biomedicine. MXenes, one of these developing 2D materials, have garnered significant attention due to their distinctive properties and promising capabilities in biomedical applications. MXenes, a class of 2D transition metal carbides, nitrides, and carbonitrides first identified in 2011, are rapidly establishing themselves as leaders in the quest for new materials. MXenes, with their exceptional electrical conductivity, mechanical flexibility, and surface chemical tunability, offer an interesting platform for addressing key challenges in biomedical engineering [1–4]. The introduction of 2D materials has sparked a resurgence in advancements within disease therapy and biomedicine. These nanomaterials exhibit superior characteristics, including enhanced performance, increased flexibility, and greater compatibility when compared to individual graphene elements [5,6]. Moreover, their ultrathin thickness and two-dimensional morphological structure impart distinctive chemical, electronic, and physical properties distinct from their larger-scale counterparts.

MXene represents a newly recognized category of two-dimensional materials. They are produced from the targeted removal through the etching of specific elements from their layered compounds with ternary nitrides/carbides characteristics, commonly referred to as MAX phases. The structure of MXene can be expressed as $M_{n+1}AX_nT_x$ (where, n = 1–3), wherein M represents transition metals as shown in Figure 1.1, A denotes main-group elements, primarily from the 13 and 14 groups, and X represents carbon/nitrogen constituents. T signifies surface termination groups found

DOI: 10.1201/9781003353287-1

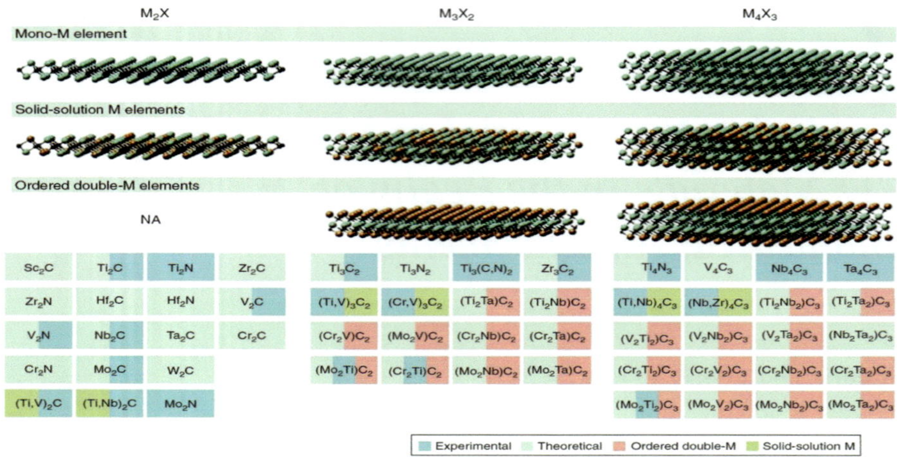

FIGURE 1.1
Classification of MXenes [10].

on MXene, which encompass fluorine, oxygen, chlorine, and hydroxyl. Meanwhile, x denotes the quantity of surface functionalities present on these materials [7–9].

MXene-based materials show various electronic, structural, optical, elastic, thermoelectric, magnetic, and dielectric properties [11]. Because of its versatile properties, it makes several compounds in varying dimensions. The detailed discussion about MXene, different synthesis methods, and properties have already reviewed in our previous work. This chapter mainly focuses on the biomedical advancements of MXene and MXene-based materials.

The unique combination of properties exhibited by MXenes opens up avenues for innovation in biomedical engineering [12]. MXene-based materials provide a unique set of properties, which includes a larger surface area, outstanding electrical conductivity, mechanical flexibility, and changeable surface chemistry [13]. These features offer researchers a diverse platform for finding novel answers to long-standing biomedical difficulties such as disease diagnosis, treatment, and regenerative medicine [14,15]. MXenes can combine various capabilities onto a single material substrate, allowing the creation of multifunctional biomedical devices and systems. Researchers develop unique solutions that outperform existing methodologies in terms of performance, efficiency, and versatility by combining qualities such as biosensing, drug administration, and tissue regeneration on a single platform.

The varied characteristics and capabilities of MXene-based materials continue to spur inquiry and discovery in new fields of biological research. From wearable devices for remote health monitoring to organ-on-a-chip systems for testing drugs and disease modeling, MXene-based technologies are pushing the boundaries of biomedicine and driving innovation across several fields [16]. In general, the promise for innovation in MXene-based biomedical applications stems from their distinct features, multifunctional capabilities, targeted therapies, personalized medicine methods, new applications, and collaborative research initiatives. Using these capabilities, researchers may create breakthrough technologies and solutions to solve unmet medical needs, enhance patient outcomes, and impact the future of health care.

This introductory chapter sets the groundwork for investigating the wide range of biomedical applications provided by MXenes. Throughout this book, we will explore the multifaceted nature of MXene-based materials and their revolutionary impact in a plethora of significant fields, including bioimaging, biosensing, therapeutic agents, tissue engineering, and more.

The demand for this book emanates from growing awareness and ability of MXene-based materials for transforming biological research and health care. As the field of materials science progresses, there is a great demand for comprehensive sources that explore the various applications, features, and ramifications of MXenes in medicine. This book serves as a pertinent and important resource for researchers, engineers, doctors, and students seeking to better understand the unique characteristics of MXene-based materials and their prospective influence on health care. The present work fills a major vacuum in the literature by providing an in-depth account of MXene-based biomedical applications spanning from biosensing and tissue engineering to drug delivery and regenerative medicine. It also promotes knowledge transfer, collaboration, and innovation in the field. Furthermore, as the field of MXene-based materials rapidly evolves, this book serves as a foundation for future research efforts, directing researchers toward discoveries, applications, and translational opportunities in biomedical science and engineering. Subsequently, the importance of this book derives from its ability to stimulate advances in health care by leveraging the revolutionary potential of MXene-based materials to alleviate medical gaps, improve patient outcomes, and improve the quality of life for people all over the world.

1.2 Synthesis Methods

MXenes are produced by processing their MAX phase counterparts, involving the disruption of the M-A (metal type) connection through an etching process that removes the A constituent. The selective etching method is influenced by various factors, including the concentration and type of the etchant, as well as the temperature, duration, and environmental conditions during the etching process. The conditions necessary for etching vary based on the type of MAX precursor being utilized. The choice of the elemental component to be removed and the energy required to break the M-A bond (for exfoliation

TABLE 1.1

Different Methods of Etchings Based on the Application with their Advantages and Limitations

S. no.	Synthesis method	Etchants used	Applications	Advantages	Limitations
1.	Hydrofluoric acid (HF) etching method	HF	Biomedical applications	This conventional approach to synthesizing MXene is widely adopted due to its highly effective performance. It is a cost-effective and straightforward method that also provides a high yield of the product	Because of the significant toxicity associated with HF, this method poses environmental hazards. Therefore, it is advisable to refrain from using this method due to its adverse ecological impact
2.	In situ HF etching	LiF + HCl with HF	EMI shielding	This method reduces potential risks and is significantly more environmentally friendly compared to traditional methods. High-quality MXene can be achieved through the in situ HF etching method	The reported data indicate that higher concentrations of HF are hazardous and corrosive. Therefore, it is recommended to avoid this method
3.	Lewis acid molten salt etching	HCl/LiF (fluoride salt with Lewis acid) and HF	EMI shielding, wound healing, etc.	Having nearly single terminations, this method is convenient to use. It also decreases the amount of liquid waste disposal and associated difficulties	This method necessitates higher temperatures for synthesis, exceeding 600°C. Consequently, it is not considered environmentally friendly
4.	Modified acid etching method	Combination of fluoride salts like LiF, NaF, KF, FeF_3 and NH_4HF_2 + HCl	Biomedical applications like tissue engineering, drug delivery, biosensors, etc.	This method is more convenient than the above ones and is also reported as excellently efficient	High concentrations of chemicals may be harmful to the environment
5.	Electrochemical etching	Electrodes	Environmental applications like OER, HER	An organized and systematic approach offers a safe and cost-effective means of synthesizing MXene. Moreover, it stands out for its non-toxic properties, distinguishing it from other methods	This method exhibits over-etching tendencies and is characterized by low efficiency
6.	Molten fluoride salt etching method	Salts of molten fluoride CsF, NaF, tetrabutylammonium fluoride $[(C_4H_9)_4NF]$, CaF_2 and KF	Supercapacitors, energy-storage materials	Employing mild etchants guarantees minimal pinholes or defects in the product, while also being less toxic compared to previously described methods	The amount of yield obtained from this route is less and the route is also difficult

Source: [17].

purposes) determine the chemical etchant used in the exfoliation process. Based on the application, different etching methods are available. Table 1.1 gives us a brief overview of the different techniques of etching used for the synthesis of MXene, and various kind of etchants used there with their advantages and limitations.

1.3 The Promise of MXenes in Biomedical Applications

Due to their distinctive characteristics, MXenes hold great potential to transform several areas of clinical practice and biological research. They are excellent candidates for biological system interfaces because of their high surface area and good biocompatibility, which could lead to breakthroughs in regenerative medicine, therapies, and diagnostics [18]. This work is organized to offer a thorough examination of materials based on MXene in biological applications. The following chapters focus on a particular area where MXenes show great promise. The chapters that follow will discuss on:

MXenes' outstanding electrical capabilities create highly sensitive biosensors able to detect a broad spectrum of analytes with unprecedented precision and efficiency. MXenes have excellent optical characteristics, making them interesting candidates for bioimaging applications. Their capacity to absorb and emit light across a wide range of wavelengths makes them suitable for utilization as contrast agents across various imaging modalities, such as photoacoustic imaging, fluorescence imaging, and optical imaging. They are used to change medical imaging procedures, allowing for improved molecular visibility and diagnosis. By using MXene-based electrodes, it is helpful to detect and quantify biomarkers, enabling early illness diagnosis along with personalized therapy techniques. MXenes have photothermal properties that can be used for therapeutic purposes, such as photothermal therapy for cancer treatment, providing a non-invasive and extremely effective approach to tumor ablation. MXenes' potential for creating biomimetic scaffolds for tissue regeneration and organ-on-a-chip applications is being investigated, to transform the area of regenerative medicine. Integrating MXene-based materials with wearable devices will enable real-time health monitoring, ushering in a new era of personalized healthcare solutions. MXenes are being investigated as drug-delivery vehicles and theragnostic platforms, which will allow for precise drug targeting and therapeutic efficacy monitoring. The regenerative capabilities of MXene can be used to stimulate tissue repair and regeneration, providing new treatment options for severe injuries and degenerative diseases. Furthermore, MXenes have been demonstrated to have antibacterial and antimicrobial properties that can be used to treat bacterial infections and

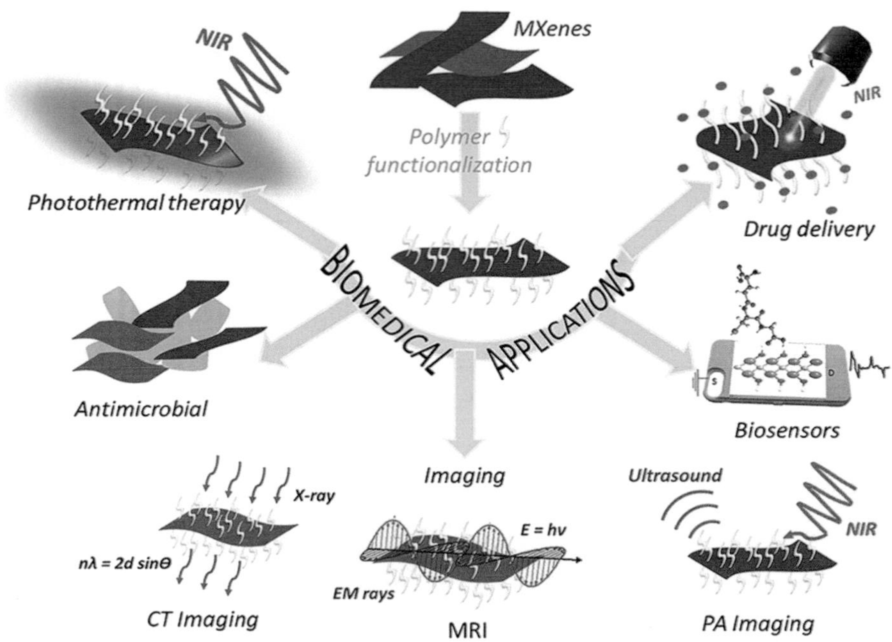

FIGURE 1.2
Role of MXenes in advancing biomedical technology [19].

prevent microbial colonization of surfaces. MXenes and their derivatives can be used to combat the growing threat of antibiotic resistance and nosocomial infections. Their capacity to prevent bacterial growth and biofilm formation makes them excellent candidates for producing antimicrobial coatings, wound dressings, and medical implants that are more resistant to bacterial infections. MXenes are also being investigated for their function in expediting wound-healing processes, to develop new wound dressings with improved antibacterial and regenerative capabilities. Each chapter will provide a complete review of current cutting-edge research, highlighting major advances, difficulties, and future prospects in the relevant topic (Figure 1.2).

1.4 Critical Properties of MXene: Key Factors Driving Biomedical Potential

MXenes possess a variety of unique properties that are especially relevant to biomedical applications. These features include a large surface area, superior electrical conductivity, mechanical flexibility, and variable surface chemistry. These attributes are ideal for interacting with biological systems and building biomedical devices. The distinct properties of MXene refer to certain characteristics that distinguish these materials from others and make them very appealing for a variety of applications, including biomedical applications. Some of the distinctive characteristics of MXene include those described in the following subsections.

1.4.1 High Surface Area and Excellent Electrical Conductivity

MXenes typically have a large surface area due to their layered structure, which consists of atomically thin sheets piled on top of one another. MXenes are useful for adsorption, sensing, and catalysis because of their large surface area, which allows for numerous interactions with molecules, cells, or other materials [20,21]. MXenes are known for their high electrical conductivity, which is due to their metallic composition. This feature permits efficient electron transport, making MXenes ideal for use in electronic devices, sensors, and energy-storage applications. Their remarkable electrical conductivity and surface chemical tunability make them ideal for developing biosensing systems with high sensitivity, selectivity, and response time.

1.4.2 Mechanical Flexibility

MXenes are mechanically flexible, considering their thin and layered structure [22]. This versatility enables MXene-based materials to conform to varied surfaces or deform without losing structural integrity, which is useful for applications that require flexibility or robustness, such as flexible electronics or wearable devices. MXene-based materials can be included in wearable devices to provide continuous monitoring of physiological parameters in real time such as heart rate, temperature, and glucose levels. Their electrical conductivity, mechanical flexibility, and biocompatibility make them ideal for creating wearable sensors and electrodes that can adjust to the body's contours and sustain long-term use in dynamic situations [23]. MXene-based wearable devices have the potential to revolutionize remote health monitoring, fitness tracking, and tailored medication.

MXene-based materials also hold potential for tissue engineering applications, as they can be used to create scaffolds or matrices that promote tissue regeneration and repair. Their mechanical flexibility, biocompatibility, and surface chemical tunability make them optimal for promoting proliferation, cell adhesion, and differentiation. MXene-based scaffolds have the potential to construct functioning tissues and organs for transplantation and regenerative medicine. They can cause localized hyperthermia to eliminate cancer cells while sparing surrounding healthy tissues by selectively absorbing near-infrared light and turning it into heat.

1.4.3 Biocompatibility

MXenes have been discovered to be extremely biocompatible, which means they are well tolerated by living beings and with less notable side effects. This feature is critical for biomedical applications since it reduces toxicity and enhances compatibility with biological systems, making MXenes appropriate for use in drug-delivery systems, medical devices, and tissue engineering scaffolds [24]. Biocompatibility refers to a material's capacity to interact with biological systems, such as live tissues or organisms, without causing detrimental consequences or undesirable reactions. Biocompatibility is an important factor in biomedical applications since it has a direct impact on the safety and effectiveness of medical devices, implants, drug-delivery systems, and other biomaterials [25]. Biocompatibility is a complicated quality that is affected by several elements, including the material's chemical composition, surface characteristics, structure, and mechanical qualities, as well as the biological environment in which it will be utilized [26].

MXene-based materials prevent side effects such as inflammation, immunological responses, and tissue damage. They are intended to be inert or barely reactive in the biological environment [3,12]. These materials are frequently developed to resemble the qualities of natural tissues, reducing the chance of immune detection. They are consistent with biological processes such as adhesion, proliferation, differentiation, and migration [27]. This assures that the material will merge seamlessly with the surrounding biological tissues and perform the appropriate physiological activities. When implanted or employed in biological contexts, these materials preserve structural integrity and functionality for an extended period.

1.4.4 Tunable Surface Chemistry

One of the foremost striking features that differentiates MXenes is their changeable surface chemistry. Surface functionalization, for example, can improve biocompatibility, provide targeted ligands for drug administration, or allow biomolecules to be immobilized for biosensing applications.

MXene-based nanosheets are capable of doing so by using various surface functionalization processes to impart certain traits or capabilities, such as increased biocompatibility, targeted drug delivery, or better cellular interactions [28]. It is the ability to adjust and regulate the chemical composition and properties of a material's surface. This often involves surface functionalization, i.e., the introduction of functional groups, molecules, or nanoparticles to the surface of a material. These alterations can be made by a variety of chemical, physical, or biological mechanisms, including covalent bonding, adsorption, and electrostatic interactions. The biocompatibility of the materials is improved by changing the surface qualities of a material by selectively adding different functional groups, such as hydrophilicity, charge, wettability, or reactivity [12,29].

Functionalizing the surfaces of a biomaterial with biocompatible chemicals or polymers can reduce non-specific protein adsorption, lessen immunological reactions, and improve positive interactions with biological tissues or cells. This is especially crucial in drug-delivery systems, medical implants, and tissue engineering scaffolds, where biocompatibility is essential [30]. MXene-based materials also permit the development of medication-delivery systems with precise targeting capabilities. They can selectively target sick tissues or cells while limiting off-target effects by adding targeting ligands, such as antibodies or peptides, to the surface of nanoparticles or microparticles.

Apart from the above-mentioned properties, MXenes offer versatility in terms of their potential applications in biomedicine. They find utility in a myriad of biomedical applications, encompassing bioimaging, biosensing, drug delivery, tissue engineering, and therapies. This adaptability underlines MXenes' potential for enhancing scientific research and therapeutic treatment.

MXene-based materials have a large spectrum of characteristics, rendering them appropriate across a range of biomedical applications. These materials can be designed to meet specific difficulties and requirements in a variety of biomedical sectors, including diagnostics, treatments, regenerative medicine, and bioengineering [31]. MXene-based materials can be used to create very sensitive biosensors that detect a variety of biological analytes, including biomarkers and infections. MXene-based contrast agents provide improved imaging capabilities for observing biological structures and processes at high resolution and sensitivity. They are designed to act as carriers for therapeutic agents like medicines or nucleic acids, allowing for targeted delivery to specific tissues or cells. Their vast surface area and adjustable surface chemistry allow for effective loading and regulated release of therapeutic payloads, increasing the efficacy and safety of drug-delivery systems. MXene-based drug carriers have potential applications in cancer treatment, gene therapy, and regenerative medicine [32].

The adaptability of MXene-based materials is due to their unique combination of characteristics, facilitating them to be applied across a broad range of biomedical applications. MXenes provide promising potential for transforming health care through innovative technologies and solutions, including biosensing and bioimaging, medication delivery, tissue engineering, and more.

1.5 Significance of Specific Application Areas

1.5.1 Biosensing

Biosensing is the detection and measurement of biological molecules or analytes such as proteins, DNA, or tiny molecules for use in diagnostics, environmental monitoring, and biomedical research. MXene-based biosensors provide numerous benefits, including high sensitivity, fast reaction times, and compatibility with complicated biological samples. The importance of biosensing stems from its capacity to offer precise and timely information on disease biomarkers, viruses, or environmental toxins, allowing for early detection, disease monitoring, and individualized healthcare interventions [33,34].

1.5.2 Bioimaging/Diagnostic Imaging

Bioimaging refers to a variety of imaging techniques used to visualize biological structures, processes, and activities on a cellular or molecular level. MXene-based contrast agents and imaging probes improve imaging capabilities for techniques like optical imaging, computed tomography (CT), magnetic resonance imaging (MRI), and fluorescence imaging. Bioimaging is important because it can provide precise insights into illness progression, treatment response, and physiological processes, allowing for earlier diagnosis, treatment planning, and disease monitoring [35].

1.5.3 Biomarkers

Biomarkers are quantitative indicators of biological processes, disease states, or pharmacological reactions that may be discovered and quantified to aid in diagnosis or prognosis. MXene-based electrodes detect biomarkers sensitively and selectively, allowing for the speedy and accurate diagnosis of cancer, cardiovascular illness, and infectious disorders. Biomarkers are important because they can enhance patient outcomes by aiding early illness detection, evaluating treatment response, and guiding individualized therapeutic approaches [36].

1.5.4 Photothermal Therapy

Photothermal therapy (PTT) is a minimally invasive treatment technique that uses light-absorbing materials to generate heat and selectively eliminate unhealthy cells, such as malignant tumors. MXene-based photothermal agents have significant light absorption in the near-infrared region, allowing for precision and targeted thermal ablation of malignancies while sparing adjacent healthy tissues. The relevance of PTT stems from its ability to give a non-invasive and effective therapy alternative for cancer patients, with few side effects and enhanced therapeutic outcomes [37,38].

1.5.5 Tissue Engineering

Tissue engineering is the process of creating biomimetic scaffolds or matrices that promote cell adhesion, proliferation, and differentiation for the regeneration or repair of damaged tissues and organs. MXene-based materials have distinct advantages, including mechanical flexibility, biocompatibility, and surface chemical tunability, making them ideal for creating tissue engineering scaffolds with specific features and functionalities. The importance of tissue engineering stems from its ability to address key healthcare concerns such as organ shortages, traumatic injuries, and degenerative diseases by providing alternate techniques to tissue regeneration and transplantation [39].

1.5.6 Wearable Device Applications

Wearable devices are wearable technologies that monitor physiological parameters, track activity levels, and offer real-time health monitoring for applications such as fitness tracking, disease management, and remote patient monitoring. MXene-based materials have high electrical conductivity, mechanical flexibility, and biocompatibility, making them ideal for creating wearable sensors and electrodes that fit the body's contours and can sustain repeated use [40]. Wearable device applications have the potential to encourage proactive healthcare management, facilitate early intervention, and enhance patient outcomes through continuous monitoring and individualized feedback.

1.5.7 Therapeutic Agents

Therapeutic agents, such as medicines, gene therapies, or biologics, treat diseases and improve patient outcomes by focusing on specific cellular pathways or molecular targets [15]. MXene-based polymers can be used as therapeutic agent carriers, allowing for targeted distribution, controlled release, and increased efficacy while reducing systemic toxicity. The importance of therapeutic agents stems from their ability to change disease treatment by offering focused and individualized therapeutic interventions that reduce side effects, improve drug efficacy, and improve patient compliance [41].

1.5.8 Tissue Regeneration

Tissue regeneration is the repair or replacement of damaged or diseased tissues by stimulating endogenous repair processes or transplanting foreign cells or tissues [24]. MXene-based materials have distinct features such as mechanical flexibility, biocompatibility, and surface chemical tunability, which facilitate cell adhesion, proliferation, and differentiation for tissue regeneration applications [42,43]. The significance of tissue regeneration stems from its ability to solve key healthcare requirements such as catastrophic injuries, chronic wounds, and degenerative diseases by offering alternate techniques to tissue repair and regeneration.

1.5.9 Antibacterial/Antimicrobial Properties

MXene-based materials have antibacterial and antimicrobial capabilities, which means they can impede the growth and proliferation of bacteria or other microorganisms, making them interesting candidates for use in infection management, wound healing, and antimicrobial coatings [44]. The significance of MXene-based antibacterial characteristics stems from their ability to combat antibiotic resistance, reduce nosocomial infections, and enhance patient outcomes by lowering the risk of infection and facilitating recovery.

1.5.10 Wound Healing

Wound healing refers to the complicated biological processes that occur in reaction to tissue injury, resulting in the restoration of tissue integrity and function [45]. MXene-based materials can aid in wound healing through a variety of processes, including antibacterial action, regulation of inflammatory responses, and tissue regeneration. The importance of wound healing stems from its ability to improve patient outcomes, lower healthcare costs, and improve quality of life by speeding up the healing process and preventing problems like infections and chronic wounds [46].

The potential of MXene-based materials to address important healthcare issues, enhance patient outcomes, and progress biomedical research and technology makes each application field of biomedicine significant. Researchers can create ground-breaking solutions that significantly affect patient care, disease detection, treatment, and healthcare delivery by utilizing the special qualities and functions of MXenes.

1.6 Future Prospects and Directions in MXene-Based Biomedical Research

MXene-based materials for biomedical applications are a rapidly developing field that has great potential to improve health care and address important issues in regenerative medicine, illness diagnostics, and treatment. Several future directions and consequences become apparent as researchers continue to investigate the special qualities and capacities of MXenes, as outlined below.

The goal of future research will be to maximize the performance and characteristics of materials based on MXene for certain biomedical uses. This entails optimizing surface chemistry, creating nanoscale structures, and investigating cutting-edge synthesis techniques to improve functionality, stability, and biocompatibility. The development of multifunctional MXene-based platforms that combine several functions, including drug delivery, tissue engineering, and biosensing, into a single material system is gaining popularity. These platforms provide biomedical applications with increased adaptability, effectiveness, and utility, opening the door for creative solutions to difficult healthcare problems. The creation of materials based on MXenes has enormous potential to enhance targeted drug delivery and therapy while reducing side effects. Future studies will concentrate on improving therapeutic efficacy, payload capacity, and targeting specificity to facilitate personalized and precision medicine methods for a range of illnesses, such as inflammatory disorders, cancer, and infectious diseases. MXene-based materials have significant potential for applications in regenerative medicine that involve tissue regeneration and repair. To solve pressing healthcare requirements such as organ shortages and traumatic injuries, future directions will investigate their usage in the development of biomimetic scaffolds, bioactive coatings, and cell transport systems for tissue engineering, wound healing, and organ regeneration.

For a variety of biomedical imaging modalities, MXene-based contrast agents and imaging probes provide improved imaging capabilities. With implications for improving patient outcomes and healthcare delivery, future research will concentrate on enhancing imaging sensitivity, resolution, and specificity to facilitate early illness detection, treatment monitoring, and image-guided therapies. It is expected that new and developing applications in biomedicine will arise as the field of MXene-based materials continues to develop. These could include cutting-edge methods for delivering targeted therapies, point-of-care diagnostics, theranostic platforms, and wearable medical technology. These could have a profound impact on patient management and healthcare delivery.

The conversion of laboratory findings into clinical applications is a significant problem in the realm of MXene-based biomedical materials. With implications for advancing healthcare innovation and enhancing patient care, future research efforts will concentrate on addressing regulatory and safety concerns, optimizing scalability and reproducibility, and carrying out preclinical and clinical studies to validate the efficacy and safety of MXene-based technologies. The prospects and consequences of MXene-based materials in biomedicine are wide-ranging and complex, presenting stimulating chances to improve health care via multidisciplinary research, teamwork, and innovation.

1.7 Conclusion

The exploration of MXene-based materials for biomedical applications offers a compelling narrative of innovation and potential in the realm of health care. Throughout this chapter, we have discussed MXenes' unique features and diverse capabilities, emphasizing their importance in a variety of biomedical domains. MXene-based materials have the potential to address major healthcare concerns while enhancing outcomes in a diverse range of applications, including bioimaging, biosensing, targeted medicines, and tissue regeneration. Looking ahead, prospective research objectives and consequences highlight MXenes' transformative potential for healthcare delivery, illness diagnostics, treatment, and regenerative medicine. By implementing the multidisciplinary integration of materials science, nanotechnology, and biomedical engineering, researchers can explore new horizons of innovation and transform laboratory findings into clinical applications, ultimately improving people's quality of life and well-being around the world. As we continue on this path of discovery and translation, the extraordinary potential of MXene-based materials in biomedicine encourages collaboration, research, and the pursuit of excellence in transforming health care for the benefit of society.

References

1. Fiori G, Bonaccorso F, Iannaccone G, Palacios T, Neumaier D, Seabaugh A, et al. Electronics based on two-dimensional materials. Nature Nanotechnology 2014;9:768–79.
2. Nicolosi V, Chhowalla M, Kanatzidis MG, Strano MS, Coleman JN. Liquid exfoliation of layered materials. Science (80) 2013;340:1226419.
3. Ferrari AC, Bonaccorso F, Fal'Ko V, Novoselov KS, Roche S, Bøggild P, et al. Science and technology roadmap for graphene, related two-dimensional crystals, and hybrid systems. Nanoscale 2015;7:4598–810.
4. Akinwande D, Petrone N, Hone J. Two-dimensional flexible nanoelectronics. Nature Communications 2014;5:1–12.
5. Cepellotti A, Fugallo G, Paulatto L, Lazzeri M, Mauri F, Marzari N. Phonon hydrodynamics in two-dimensional materials. Nature Communications 2015;6:1–7.
6. Xia F, Wang H, Xiao D, Dubey M, Ramasubramaniam A. Two-dimensional material nanophotonics. Nature Photonics 2014;8:899–907.
7. Xie Y, Naguib M, Mochalin VN, Barsoum MW, Gogotsi Y, Yu X, et al. Role of surface structure on Li-ion energy storage capacity of two-dimensional transition-metal carbides. Journal of the American Chemical Society 2014;136:6385–94.
8. Deysher G, Shuck CE, Hantanasirisakul K, Frey NC, Foucher AC, Maleski K, et al. Synthesis of Mo4VAlC4 MAX phase and two-dimensional Mo4VC4 MXene with five atomic layers of transition metals. American Chemical Society Nano 2019;14:204–17.
9. Hong L, Guo R, Yuan Y, Ji X, Li Z, Lin Z, et al. Recent progress of two-dimensional MXenes in photocatalytic applications: A review. Materials Today Energy 2020;18:100521.
10. Anasori B, Lukatskaya MR, Gogotsi Y. 2D metal carbides and nitrides (MXenes) for energy storage. Nature Reviews Materials 2017;2:1–17.

11. Chaturvedi K, Hada V, Paul S, Sarma B, Malvi D, Dhangar M, Bajpai H, Singhwane A, Srivastava AK, Verma S. The rise of MXene: A wonder 2D material, from its synthesis and properties to its versatile applications—A comprehensive review. Topics in Current Chemistry 2023 Mar;381(2):11.
12. Huang R, Chen X, Dong Y, Zhang X, Wei Y, Yang Z, et al. MXene composite nanofibers for cell culture and tissue engineering. ACS Applied Bio Materials 2020;3:2125–31.
13. Rakhi RB, Nayak P , Xia C, Alshareef HN. Erratum: Novel amperometric glucose biosensor based on MXene nanocomposite. Scientific Reports 2016;6.
14. Pan S, Yin J, Yu L, Zhang C, Zhu Y, Gao Y, et al. 2D MXene-integrated 3D-printing scaffolds for augmented osteosarcoma phototherapy and accelerated tissue reconstruction. Advanced Science 2020;7:1901511.
15. Yang W, Lyu Q, Zhao J, Cao L, Hao Y, Zhang H. Recent advance in near-infrared/ultrasound-sensitive 2D-nanomaterials for cancer therapeutics. Science China Materials 2020;63:2397–428.
16. Lei Y, Zhao W, Zhang Y, Jiang Q, He J, Baeumner AJ, et al. A MXene-based wearable biosensor system for high-performance in vitro perspiration analysis. Small 2019;15:1901190.
17. Verma S, Dwivedi U, Chaturvedi K, Kumari N, Dhangar M, Hashmi SA, Singhal R, Srivastava AK. Progress of 2D MXenes based composites for efficient electromagnetic interference shielding applications: A review. Synthetic Metals 2022 Jul 1;287:117095.
18. Gan W, Shang X, Li X-H, Zhang J, Fu X. Achieving high adsorption capacity and ultrafast removal of methylene blue and Pb2+ by graphene-like TiO2@ C. Colloids and Surfaces A: Physicochemical and Engineering Aspects 2019;561:218–25.
19. George SM, Kandasubramanian B. Advancements in MXene-Polymer composites for various biomedical applications. Ceramics International 2020 May 1;46(7):8522–35.
20. Tang Q, Sun Z, Deng S, Wang H, Wu Z. Decorating g-C3N4 with alkalinized Ti3C2 MXene for promoted photocatalytic CO2 reduction performance. Journal of Colloid and Interface Science 2020;564:406–17. https://doi.org/10.1016/j.jcis.2019.12.091.
21. Thanh Q, Ta H, Tran NM, Noh J. Rice Crust-Like ZnO / Ti_3C_2T. Catalysts 2020;10(10):1140.
22. Ren CE, Hatzell KB, Alhabeb M, Ling Z, Mahmoud KA, Gogotsi Y. Charge- and size-selective ion sieving through $Ti_3C_2T_x$ MXene membranes. The Journal of Physical Chemistry Letters 2015;6:4026–31.
23. Miao M, Liu R, Thaiboonrod S, Shi L, Cao S, Zhang J, et al. Silver nanowires intercalating $Ti_3C_2T_x$ MXene composite films with excellent flexibility for electromagnetic interference shielding. Journal of Materials Chemistry 2020;8:3120–6.
24. Lin X, Li Z, Qiu J, Wang Q, Wang J, Zhang H, et al. Fascinating MXene nanomaterials: Emerging opportunities in the biomedical field. Biomaterials Science 2021;9:5437–71.
25. Xie Z, Chen S, Duo Y, Zhu Y, Fan T, Zou Q, et al. Biocompatible two-dimensional titanium nanosheets for multimodal imaging-guided cancer theranostics. ACS Applied Materials & Interfaces 2019;11:22129–40.

26. Dai C, Lin H, Xu G, Liu Z, Wu R, Chen Y. Biocompatible 2D titanium carbide (MXenes) composite nanosheets for pH-responsive MRI-guided tumor hyperthermia. Chemistry of Materials 2017;29:8637–52.
27. Hou R, Wu L, Wang J, Yang Z, Tu Q, Zhang X, et al. Surface-degradable drug-eluting stent with anticoagulation, antiproliferation, and endothelialization functions. Biomolecules 2019;9:69.
28. Liu G, Zou J, Tang Q, Yang X, Zhang Y, Zhang Q, et al. Surface modified Ti_3C_2 MXene nanosheets for tumor targeting photothermal/photodynamic/chemo synergistic therapy. ACS Applied Materials & Interfaces 2017;9:40077–86.
29. Zhu J, Ha E, Zhao G, Zhou Y, Huang D, Yue G, et al. Recent advance in MXenes: A promising 2D material for catalysis, sensor and chemical adsorption. Coordination Chemistry Reviews 2017;352:306–27.
30. Wang X, Jin J , Hou R, Zhou M, Mou X, Xu K, et al. Differentiation of bMSCs on biocompatible, biodegradable, and biomimetic scaffolds for largely defected tissue repair. ACS Applied Bio Materials 2019;3:735–46.
31. Liu Y, Han Q, Yang W, Gan X, Yang Y, Xie K, et al. Two-dimensional MXene/cobalt nanowire heterojunction for controlled drug delivery and chemo-photothermal therapy. Materials Science and Engineering C 2020;116:111212.
32. Zhang H, Wang Z, Zhang Q, Wang F, Liu Y. Ti_3C_2 MXenes nanosheets catalyzed highly efficient electrogenerated chemiluminescence biosensor for the detection of exosomes. Biosensors and Bioelectronics 2019;124:184–90.
33. Sinha A, Zhao H, Huang Y, Lu X, Chen J, Jain R. MXene: An emerging material for sensing and biosensing. TrAC Trends Anal Chem 2018;105:424–35.
34. Wu L, Lu X, Wu Z-S, Dong Y, Wang X, Zheng S, et al. 2D transition metal carbide MXene as a robust biosensing platform for enzyme immobilization and ultrasensitive detection of phenol. Biosensors and Bioelectronics 2018;107:69–75.
35. Huang M, Gu Z, Zhang J, Zhang D, Zhang H, Yang Z, Qu J. MXene and black phosphorus based 2D nanomaterials in bioimaging and biosensing: Progress and perspectives. Journal of Materials Chemistry B 2021;9(26):5195–220.
36. Kumar S, Lei Y, Alshareef NH, Quevedo-Lopez MA, Salama KN. Biofunctionalized two-dimensional Ti_3C_2 MXenes for ultrasensitive detection of cancer biomarker. Biosensors and Bioelectronics 2018 Dec 15;121:243–9.
37. Wang J, Xuan J, Liu Y, Li Z, Han Y, Wang Z. NIR-dependent photothermal-photodynamic synergistic antibacterial mechanism for titanium carbide nanosheets intercalated and delaminated by tetramethylammonium hydroxide. Biomaterials Advances 2023 Jun 6:213492.
38. Liu X, Xie H, Zhuo S, Zhou Y, Selim MS, Chen X, Hao Z. Ru(II) complex grafted $Ti_3C_2T_x$ MXene nano sheet with photothermal/photodynamic synergistic antibacterial activity. Nanomaterials 2023;13:958. https://doi.org/10.3390/nano13060958
39. Basara G, Saeidi-Javash M, Ren X, Bahcecioglu G, Wyatt BC, Anasori B, Zhang Y, Zorlutuna P. Electrically conductive 3D printed Ti3C2T MXene-PEG composite constructs for cardiac tissue engineering. Acta Biomaterialia 2020:S1742706120307479. https://doi.org/10.1016/j.actbio.2020.12.033
40. Li M, Zhang Y, Lian L, Liu K, Lu M, Chen Y, Zhang L, Zhang X, Wan P. Flexible accelerated-wound-healing antibacterial MXene-based epidermic sensor for intelligent wearable human-machine interaction. Advanced Functional Materials 2022 Nov;32(47):2208141.

41. Han X, Jing X, Yang D, Lin H, Wang Z, Ran H, et al. Therapeutic mesopore construction on 2D Nb2C MXenes for targeted and enhanced chemo-photothermal cancer therapy in NIR-II biowindow. Theranostics 2018;8:4491.
42. Mayerberger EA, Street RM, McDaniel RM, Barsoum MW, Schauer CL. Antibacterial properties of electrospun $Ti_3C_2T_z$ (MXene)/chitosan nanofibers. RSC Advances 2018;8:35386–94.
43. Zhou L, Zheng H, Liu Z, Wang S, Liu Z, Chen F, et al. Conductive antibacterial hemostatic multifunctional scaffolds based on $Ti_3C_2T_x$ MXene nanosheets for promoting multidrug-resistant bacteria-infected wound healing. American Chemical Society Nano 2021;15:2468–80.
44. Singhwane A, Chaturvedi K, Mohapatra RK, Srivastava AK, Verma S. Mxene-based composite materials as antibacterial agents for healthcare applications. In Age of MXenes, Volume 2. Applications in Diagnostics, Therapeutics, and Environmental Remediation 2023. American Chemical Society, 2023, pp. 1–17.
45. Sun L, Fan L, Bian F, Chen G, Wang Y, Zhao Y. MXene-integrated microneedle patches with innate molecule encapsulation for wound healing. Research 2021; 30 Jun 2021. Article ID: 9838490. DOI: 10.34133/2021/9838490.
46. Xu X, Wang S, Wu H, Liu Y, Xu F, Zhao J. A multimodal antimicrobial platform based on MXene for treatment of wound infection. Colloids and Surfaces B: Biointerfaces 2021;207:111979.

2

MXene-Based 2D Materials for Biosensing

M. Chandrashekhar Nayak and Kajal Yadav

2.1 Introduction

MXenes are the family of two-dimensional layered materials, i.e., transition metal carbonitrides, carbides, or nitrides added to 2D nanomaterials. MXenes gain noteworthy attention in well-known scientific and industrial communities due to their unique possessions such as single-layered morphology, abundant surface area, magnetic conductance, superb hydrophilic property, respectable thermal strength, amazing electrical conductivity assets, and eco-friendly features [1]. These days, MXenes are converted as favorable aspirants in various applications, including the environment, electro-catalysis, energy storage requests, sensing drive, etc. [2,3]. Generally, and as standard, biosensors are made up of two major components: a transducer and a receptor. To date, numerous research reports can be found on MXene-based nanocomposites' engagement with biosensing ability. From the conclusions of previous research findings, MXenes with titanium carbide mixed terminations engagement are highly suitable for applications of biosensing. Functional groups on the surface of MXene –OH, –O, –F, and –Cl are exposed as very active sites and effectively form bonding interactions with nearby sites in the form of H-bonding, charge transfer, Van der Waals forces, etc. [4]. MXene-$Ti_3C_2T_x$ nanosheet with gold nanoparticle surface etched biosensors are further engaged in assessing the point of care (POC) for cancer screening of oncomiRs (microRNA-21 and microRNA-141).

During the COVID-19 pandemic, various biosensors were advanced and intended for identifying this coronavirus which causes severe acute respiratory syndrome (SARS-CoV-2) and other communicable infections. In 2022, M. Song synthesized novel Nb_2CT_x MXene layers and employed them to create a straightforward, label-free multiplex RNA exploration design, Forster resonance energy transfer (FRET) biosensor for quick and exact detection of SARS-CoV-2 variant (B.1.1.529/Omicron) and other transferrable

 DOI: 10.1201/9781003353287-2

viruses [5]. Advanced, easily accessible, cost-effective hybridized MXene/Pt/C/GCE (MXene 2D nanomaterial united with Pt/C) nanocomposite-based electrochemical nano-biosensors have been developed to diagnose the SARS-CoV-2 infection from nasopharyngeal swabs, serum, and saliva samples [6]. Zhang developed double-stranded 3D DNA walker technology and Clustered Regularly Interspaced Short Palindromic Repeats-12a (CRISPR-12a) assay systems and engaged a PEI-Ru@Ti3C2@AuNPs unified MXene-based electro-chemo-luminescent (ECL)-centered biosensor, to identify the RNA-dependent RNA polymerase (RdRp) gene of SARS-CoV-2 [7]. Wu and co-workers developed a fast, simple, operational, and highly sensitive recombinase-assisted real-time reverse transcription amplification (RT-RAA) assay which was developed to identify the SARS-CoV-2 nucleocapsid protein gene (N gene) sequence [8].

This chapter explores the recent advancements in the utilization of MXene-based 2D materials for bioanalytical biosensing applications. The chapter delves into the fundamental properties of MXenes that make them suitable for biosensing, and discusses the rise of MXene during the COVID pandemic, the fabrication of MXene-based biosensors, and highlights their performance in detecting different bioanalytical analytes. Additionally, we have explored the MXene-based electrochemical carcinogenic antigen biosensor and MXene-based DNA aptamer biosensor challenges and future prospects associated with the integration of MXene-based materials in bioanalytical biosensing, to provide insights into the potential avenues for further research and technological innovation in this rapidly evolving field.

2.2 Role of MXene Nanosheets in Biosensing

These days, in the biosensing arena, conventionally, MXenes have gained significant attention due to their noteworthy optical topographies, reputable biocompatibility assets, excellent surface area and volume ratios, good antifouling behavior, exceptional electrochemical properties, etc. Fluorine-free MXene nanosheets have shown ultrahigh sensitivity, selectivity, stability, low toxicity, and biocompatible properties, besides possibly boosting the enzyme motion and electron transfer in the biosensor [9]. The biodegradable, chemically stable, highly porous fluoride-free Nb_2CT_x nanosheets (2D niobium carbide MXenes)-acetylcholinesterase-based biosensors with good metallic conductivity ability, have shown sustainable outcomes in possible biosensing applications, as shown in Figure 2.1. The exceptional properties of this novel class of 2D nanomaterials, such as high thermal stability, hydrophilicity, and electrical conductivity, spacious

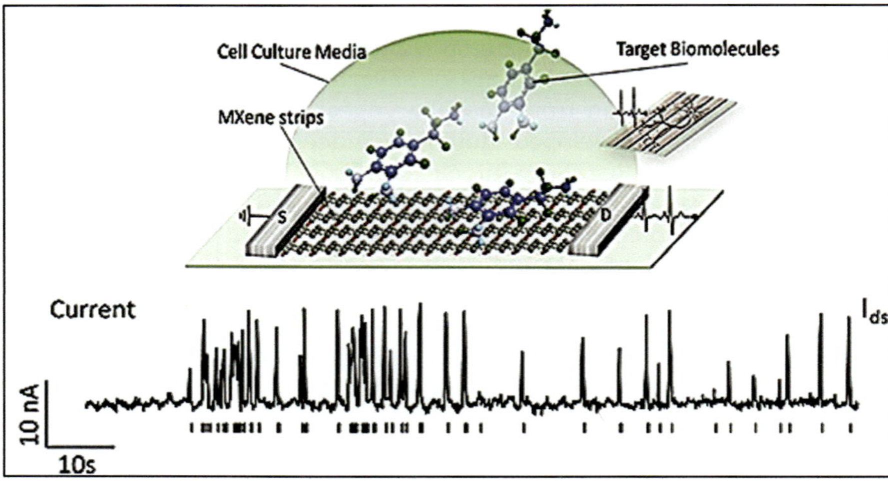

FIGURE 2.1
Diagram demonstrating underlying MXene biosensors involve alterations in the electrocatalytic properties of the MXene-based devices upon binding with target biomolecules, generating signal peaks [13].

between the layers, substantial surface area, and modifiable structure, render them highly appealing for a diverse array of applications. Due to MXenes' relatively few atomic layers, an individual MXene layer stack is generally thinner than 1 nm, and its lateral measurements range from nanometers to micrometers based on the composition, synthesis, and processing methods.

Furthermore, the choice of double-metal MXenes offers the ability to adjust relationistic spin–orbit coupling and valence states [10]. Soomro noted that keeping MXene nanosheets in vials with tight closure causes substantial degradation and oxidation, forming TiO_2 in just a few months. However, it is observed that MXene nanosheets undergoing regulated partial oxidation can present intriguing possibilities, including creating crinkled or crumpled morphologies through flocculation and enhancing the surface area. The particular experimental conditions employed will dictate the final morphology. For instance, the Willander team made use of $NiWO_4$ to induce partial oxidation of MXene for detecting prostate-specific antigens [11]. MXene sheets exhibit excellent characteristics of electrocatalysis and greater surface area. The combined influence of these two factors significantly contributed to achieving a practical limit of detection (LOD). The suggested sensor effectively detected ascorbic acid in a range of real samples, including juices and biological fluids like erythrocytes using the spiking technique, as well as serum and urine, demonstrating satisfactory performance [12].

2.3 MXenes for Bioanalytical Biosensing

Two-dimensional nanomaterials, including MoS, graphene, and boron nitride nanosheets, whether used individually or in composite structures, showcase exceptional traits as they provide expansive surface areas that are ideal for developing diverse chemical and biological sensors. Their integration into sensor designs has notably enhanced sensor performance metrics such as sensitivity, selectivity, and analyte binding. Nevertheless, challenges such as pronounced hydrophobicity, limited biocompatibility, reduced electrical conductivity, and complexities in surface functionalization pose constraints, impeding their seamless integration into sensor technologies on a commercially viable scale. Overcoming these hurdles via innovative surface modification approaches, improved biocompatibility strategies, enhanced conductivity solutions, and mitigation of hydrophobic behavior is pivotal to unleashing the full potential of these 2D nanomaterials, facilitating broader sensor applications across various industries, including health care and environmental monitoring [14].

Over the last few decades, there has been a discernible increase in interest in utilizing MXenes across various technological domains. These include their application in developing supercapacitors, transparent conductors, Li-ion batteries, hybrid nanocomposites, field-effect transistors, electromagnetic interface shields, and catalysts, as well as their use in sensors. MXenes have found significant interest in biological sensors, leveraging their attributes as an electrode material. Their utilization capitalizes on their exceptional catalytic prowess, expansive surface area, efficient charge transport properties, and compatibility with biological matrices.

2.3.1 MXene-Based Enzyme Biosensors

Enzymes are substrates, for example, biological catalysts, typically composed of proteins, that are produced by living organisms. They play a crucial role in facilitating various physiological reactions by interacting with specific substrates to generate the desired products. Currently, electrochemical biosensors are most commonly used in bio-related interactions to bind/integrate the substrate/antibody/enzyme to the target analyte, and in later stages the electrochemical (EC) signaling process continues. Due to the cost-effective, extremely effective, sensitive properties, the emerging EC biosensing technology is the most extensively used for advancing and detecting enzymatic inhibitors, etc. [15]. MXene nanocomposite utilization in enzyme-based biosensing areas is gradually growing [16]. MXene-Ti_3C_2 2D transition metal carbides have nanographene 2D structures besides the outer surface moderately concluded with –OH, thus offering a promotable microenvironment for enzyme immobilization, high sensitivity, reproducibility, durable strength, and holding bioactivity strength. It is thus further confirmed as a multipurpose enzyme- based biosensor, and depicted in biomedical research findings. The study by Kong led to nano-enzymes of Ti_3C_2 or nano-enzyme (NE) creation, exhibiting simulated quenching of fluorescence and peroxidase activity attributes. Subsequently, functionalization of Ti_3C_2 NEs was conducted by employing aptamers labeled with 6-carboxyfluorescein (FAM) and aflatoxin B1 (AFB1), thus creating an innovative optimized multi-mode nanoenzyme biosensor ready for AFB1 identification in peanuts [17]. Ghodrati introduced a biosensor using surface plasmon resonance (SPR) employing Ti_3C_2Tx MXene, a material with two dimensions, for detecting uric acid through the utilization of urate oxidase enzyme. The biosensor configuration suggested involves a free space structure utilizing the Kretschmann configuration to excite surface plasmons [18].

2.3.1.1 Hydrogen Peroxide (H_2O_2) Sensor

Hydrogen peroxide (H_2O_2) is an important antiseptic, bleaching agent, and oxidizing agent, that is regularly used in chemical reactions, food industries, medicine, biological reactions, and for ecological protection. H_2O_2 with active and reactive oxygen species (ROS) might have a short/longer life-time depending on the intensity of antioxidant enzymes. Endogenous and exogenous factors can impact the H_2O_2 attention. It interrupts the biological functions of the human body so that the oxidative stress levels may increase, and sometimes high H_2O_2 levels in the stomach may cause gastrointestinal infections. Portable, cheap, and rapid-detecting knowledge through great sensitivity is highly anticipated for the detection of H_2O_2. Mediator-free biosensors invented using a blend of TiO_2 altered with Ti_3C_2 MXene (TiO_2-Ti_3C_2) nanocomposites, have been engaged to immobilize the hemoglobin (Hb) protein matrix with biocompatibility and for the detection of stability, reproducibility, and electrochemical conduct of H_2O_2 biosensor s[19]. In 2023, Gao et al. developed a microfluidic technology that uses hydrophobic ionic liquid (HIL) coordination-aided Hb-based biosensors to detect H_2O_2. At this juncture, the employed microfluidic station acted as a Hb immobilizer in the HIL microreactor (HIL@Hb), so that it could effectively affect the Hb agglomeration. After this, the HIL@Hb electrodes are introduced to the MXene-Ti_3C_2 nanosheet surface so that the MXene-Ti_3C_2 nanosheet surface conductivity is affected, and then the electron transferability is improved, i.e., H_2O_2 sensing capacity can be improved [20]. Nanocrystal-structured iron oxide (α-Fe_2O_3) was synthesized through a solid-phase process, and further deposited on the MXene-$Ti_3C_2T_x$ nanosheet surface ($Ti_3C_2T_x$-Fe_2O_3) to assess the electro-catalytic activity for H_2O_2 reduction capability from food and urine models [21]. Tong's studies showed that an electrochemical biosensor could be created using enzyme development by using nanocomposites featuring multiple steady interface configurations, particularly PGOx@MXene/

CS nanocomposites. At the same time, the expansive MXenes' specific surface area facilitated effective nanocapsule (PGOx) loading. It catalyzed the breakdown of the hazardous intermediate H_2O_2, thereby mitigating its impact on enzyme stability [22].

2.3.1.2 Nitrite Sensor

Usually, in the food industries, the addition of nitrite (NO_2^-) to food materials is expected as it prevents food spoilage and avoids surface bacterial growth so that the food material can be preserved for a long time [23]. By directly taking this type of food into the stomach, it reacts with secondary amines and then forms teratogenic and carcinogenic nitrosamines, causing gastric and esophageal cancer, in addition to nitrites reacting with hemoglobin, causing the symptoms of methemoglobinemia disease. In recent years, researchers have been more focused on developing simple, cost-effective, less time-consuming, and more convenient electrochemical techniques. Liu produced novel graphene-like 2D layered nanosheets (MXene-Ti_3C_2), further making a mediator-free electrochemical biosensor to distinguish the nitrite (NO_2^-) detection limitations. At this stage, the model protein is hemoglobin (Hb). In the outcomes, compared with glass carbon electrode (GCE) and Nafion/Hb/MXene-Ti_3C_2/GCE, grounded biosensors showed promising outcomes in stability, reproducibility, enzyme immobilization, and electrochemical motion in identifying $NaNO_2$ [24]. Wang developed gold nanoparticles that confined poly(dimethyl diallyl ammonium chloride)-adorned MXene (Ti_3C_2Tx) (AuNPs/Ti_3C_2Tx-PDDA)-based ultrasensitive high-performance electrochemical biosensors to assess their nitrite-sensing viability. The drop-coating technique was engaged in advancing electrode materials such as $Ti_3C_2T_x$-PDDA and $Ti_3C_2T_x$-PDDA/GCE, and later Au NPs were deposited on $Ti_3C_2T_x$-PDDA/GCE by a potentiostatic deposition technique. AuNPs/Ti_3C_2Tx-PDDA/GCE contributed impressive outcomes in stability, reproducibility, and feasibility for NO_2^- detection sensitivity [25]. Wang introduced a novel nanocomposite, MXene/AuNPs/ERGO, designed for susceptible electrochemical nitrite detection. The nanocomposite was synthesized via a simple single-step electrodeposition process involving mixing MXene, $HAuCl_4$, and GO in a PBS solution for 600 seconds at an applied potential of −1.4 V [26]. A study by Feng created an electrochemical sensor that is susceptible to nitrite detection using a one-pot green synthesis approach based on electrochemical techniques. The incorporation of MXene, known for its excellent electrical conductivity, acted as an immobile matrix to create Au@CQDs-MXene nanocomposites. These nanocomposites combined the benefits of robust conductivity of electricity and electrocatalytic properties. Building an electrochemical nitrite-monitoring sensor involved the application of Au@CQDs-MXene onto a carbon electrode made of glass [27].

2.3.1.3 Glucose Sensor

Diabetes mellitus is an incurable metabolic disease; controlling blood glucose levels with continuous medication is the only way to care for diabetic patients. At present, there are many feasible and self-testing approaches, but these are quite expensive, and direct blood collection methods from diabetic patients are fairly inconvenient. Pan developed a new type of hydrogel made of conductive polymer composite, i.e., a hydrogel cross-linked MXene-based poly(3,4-ethylene-dioxythiophene) and poly(styrene sulfonate) (PEDOT:PSS) blended electrically conductive biosensing device to assess glucose levels. Hydrogels have good film-forming ability, and the films can be directly patched on the skin to diagnose diabetic patients' sugar levels directly. PEDOT:PSS/MXene/GOx/hydrogel fused screen-printed carbon electrodes (SPCEs) revealed better outcomes with glucose biosensing of the skin patch in vitro [28]. Wu technologically advanced poly-L-lysine (PLL) altered ultra-thin Ti_3C_2 MXene nanosheets (Ti_3C_2-PLL) supplementary immobilized glucose oxidase (GOx) on Ti_3C_2 MXene nanosheets (Ti_3C_2-PLL-GOx) which were then employed to assess the enzyme adsorption efficiency.

The biosensing activity of the hybrid Ti_3C_2-PLL-GOx nanosheets was examined [29] over the enzymatic oxidation of glucose by maintaining the different wt.% of GOx loadings. Ti_3C_2-PLL-GOx/GCE confined biosensors showed better electrical conductivity, stability, and favorable high performance catalytic activity for glucose detection as shown in Figure 2.2.

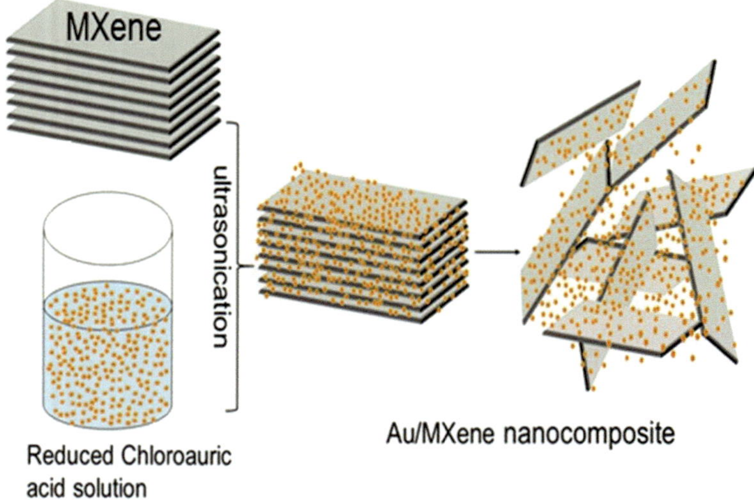

FIGURE 2.2
Preparation of (A) $Ti_3C_2T_x$ MXene nanosheets; (B) pure $Ti_3C_2T_x$ film, standalone graphene film, and the hybrid film of $Ti_3C_2T_x$ and graphene for enzyme immobilization [14].

Feng utilized a straightforward process of mixing, freezing, drying, and self-reduction to engineer three-dimensional porous composites of $Ti_3C_2T_x$ MXene/graphene/AuNPs (MGA). The abundance of $Ti_3C_2T_x$ MXene nanosheets' hydrophilic groups provides the MXene/graphene/AuNP composites with exceptionally water-attracting properties. These three-dimensional porous composites boast an open structure that facilitates the entry of glucose oxidase into their interior pore, potentially improving GOx's sustained immobilization and retention within the film. Leveraging the distinctive electrocatalytic characteristics and $Ti_3C_2T_x$ MXene/graphene synergistic effects with AuNPs, they have further elevated electron movement in the three-dimensional porous composites while simultaneously lowering redox potential. The resultant MXene/graphene/AuNPs/GOx glucose sensor exhibits a current in linear form response across a glucose concentration spectrum between 2 µM and 0.4 mM, and from 0.4 mM to 6 mM, respectively [30]. This study presents a wearable, flexible, non-enzymatic electrochemical sensor designed for continuous glucose monitoring in sweat. To achieve this, the Pt nanoparticles were combined onto MXene (Ti_3C_2Tx) nanosheets to create a catalyst (Pt/MXene). This resulted in a sensor with a wide linear glucose detection range (0–8 mmol/L) in neutral circumstances.

2.3.2 MXene-Based Electrochemical Carcinoembryonic Antigen Biosensor

In the case of many diseases, launching ultra-sensitive detectors to detect tumor markers in the early stage is challenging. Carcinoembryonic antigen (CEA) is a cancer biomarker (protein) that is mostly discovered in liver, ovarian, colorectal, pancreatic, lung, and breast cancer patients. As per a World Health Organization (WHO) 2018 report, nearly half of cancer death cases are from these cancers [32]. An alternative biosensor for CEA, based on MXene, was documented employing a sandwich-type immunoassay setup. This method involved initially functionalizing Ti_3C_2 with amino silane (APTES) to covalently immobilize monoclonal anti-carcino embryonic antigen antibodies (Ab1) detection through surface plasmon resonance. In 2022, Song etched a MXene nanosheet with trimetallic Au-Pd-Pt nanoparticles, as a catalytic sensing interface, and the modified Au-Pd-Pt/$Ti_3C_2T_x$ electrode created a sensitive, label-free, aptamer-based CEA detection monitor [33]. Wu introduced a SPR sensing technology-based early-stage CEA detector in human serum. In this process, the initially synthesized Ti_3C_2-MXene nanosheet surface was functionalized with AuNP composites and staphylococcal protein-A (SPA). Subsequently, a monoclonal anti-CEA antibody (Ab1) was immobilized via its fragment crystallizable (Fc) region, followed by the addition of MWCNTs and polydopamine. Multi-walled carbon nanotubes-polydopamine-AgNPs-polyclonal anti-CEA antibody conjugate structures provided CEA detection limits by a biosensing method and revealed good reproducibility [34]. Luo focused on creating a disposable electrode chip for electrochemiluminescence (ECL) with a screen-printed electrode to detect carcinoembryonic antigen (CEA) through ECL technology. To achieve this, a Ti_3C_2 MXene modified with amino acid was employed in the role of a carrier. This enabled the development of a very effective electrochemiluminescence probe termed AuNPs-Ru-Arg@ NH_2-Ti_3C_2-MXene. This probe was crafted by loading AuNPs-Arg using covalent bonds onto the Ti_3C_2 MXene and adding a ruthenium complex to modify it [35]. Kalkal's research focused on creating an electrochemical biosensing platform based on a nanohybrid thin film composed of f-graphene@ Ti_3C_2-MXene, aimed at detecting carcinoembryonic antigen efficiently. This method of air-brush spray coating has been employed to deposit uniformly distributed thin films of Ti_3C_2-MXene nanohybrid and amine-functionalized graphene (f-graphene) on an ITO-coated glass substrate [36]. On the other hand, Kumar introduced the creation of an exceptionally responsive electrochemical immunosensor design for directly detecting EpCAM antigen without the need for labeling [37].

2.3.3 MXene-Based DNA/Aptamer Biosensor

Bioanalytical platforms utilizing biosensors for the detection of nucleic acid and monitoring hybridization events have been extensively documented, employing optical or electrical output mechanisms [38]. In recent studies, MXenes are becoming a more viable electrode material for monitoring hybridization events and improving detection sensitivity. MXene nanosheets function as a scaffold for hosting DNA and Pd/Pt within the engineered biosensor. The molecules of DNA were initially deposited onto the surface of MXene, facilitated by the nucleotide bases' and MXene nanosheets' π–π stacking interaction. Subsequently, the production of Pd and Pt nanoparticles in situ occurs when DNA/MXene nanocomposites are present [39]. A newly developed electrochemical biosensor utilizing an AuNPs/Ti_3C_2 MXene 3D nanocomposite has been introduced for highly sensitive detection of microRNA-155, employing exonuclease III-assisted cascade target recycling [40]. Fan P synthesized an amino-functionalized few-layer $Ti_3C_2T_x$ MXene (referred to as $Ti_3C_2NH_2$ MXene) through an etching process utilizing a LiF/HCl etching mixture. Subsequently, reduced gold nanoparticles anchored onto the $Ti_3C_2NH_2$ MXene surface to produce $Ti_3C_2NH_2$ MXene@Au. This composite was employed to create an exceptionally sensitive electrically powered DNA biosensor for quick identification of HBV-DNA [41]. A study was conducted to develop an electrochemical sensor for *M. tuberculosis*, employing a particular segment of the 16S rDNA from *M. tuberculosis* H37Ra as the target biomarker. They used highly conductive two-dimensional Ti_3C_2 MXenes as the material for signal amplification in the transduction process and peptide nucleic acid (PNA) as the capture probe [42]. Wang reported a newly developed electrochemical DNA sensor that was created for the detection of *Helicobacter pylori*, utilizing accordion-like $Ti_3C_2T_x$. In this design, the glass carbon electrode was modified using multilayered $Ti_3C_2T_x$ obtained through DMSO delamination, leveraging its substantial specific surface area and superior conductivity [43].

2.4 Conclusion and Future Perspectives

MXene-based 2D materials have demonstrated immense potential and versatility in biosensing. Their exceptional properties, including high electrical conductivity, large surface area, and customizable surface chemistry, have enabled significant advancements in biosensor development. The ability to fine-tune MXene properties through surface modifications and functionalizations has enhanced their sensitivity, selectivity, and biocompatibility for detecting various biomolecules and analytes. The research thus far showcases the promising capabilities of MXenes in offering susceptible and specific biosensing platforms across diverse applications, ranging from healthcare diagnostics to environmental monitoring. However, challenges such as stability, reproducibility, and scalability warrant further investigation and refinement in MXene-based biosensing technologies.

Future directions in this field should address these challenges by exploring novel synthesis methods, optimizing surface modifications, and developing standardized protocols for biosensor fabrication. Additionally, integrating MXene-based sensors with advanced technologies, such as microfluidics or machine learning algorithms, could further enhance their performance and broaden their application scope. MXene-based 2D materials hold tremendous promise as innovative and efficient tools in biosensing, paving the way for developing highly sensitive, portable, and reliable detection platforms with significant implications in health care, biotechnology, and environmental monitoring. Continued research efforts and collaborative endeavors will be instrumental in unlocking the full potential of MXenes in revolutionizing the field of biosensing.

References

1. Naguib M, Kurtoglu M, Presser V, Lu J, Niu J, Heon M, Hultman L, Gogotsi Y, Barsoum MW. Two-dimensional nanocrystals produced by exfoliation of Ti_3AlC_2. Advanced Materials 23 (2011) 4248–4253.
2. Chaturvedi K, Hada V, Paul S, Sarma B, Malvi D, Dhangar M, Bajpai H, Singhwane A, Srivastava AK, Verma S. The rise of MXene: A wonder 2D

material, from its synthesis and properties to its versatile applications—A comprehensive review. Topics in Current Chemistry 2023 Mar;381(2):11.
3. Verma S, Dwivedi U, Chaturvedi K, Kumari N, Dhangar M, Hashmi SA, Singhal R, Srivastava AK. Progress of 2D MXenes based composites for efficient electromagnetic interference shielding applications: A review. Synthetic Metals 2022 Jul 1;287:117095.
4. Ng VMH, Huang H, Zhou K, Lee PS, Que W, Xu ZJ, Kong LB. Recent progress in layered transition metal carbides and/or nitrides (MXenes) and their composites: Synthesis and applications. Journal of Materials Chemistry A 2017;5:1192.
5. Song M, Ma Y, Li L, Wong MC, Wang P, Chen J, ... & Hao J. Multiplexed detection of SARS-CoV-2 based on upconversion luminescence nanoprobe/MXene biosensing platform for COVID-19 point-of-care diagnostics. Materials & Design 2022;223:111249.
6. Bolourinezhad M, Rezayi M, Meshkat Z, Soleimanpour S, Mojarrad M, Aghaee-Bakhtiari SH, Taghdisi SM. Design of a rapid electrochemical biosensor based on MXene/Pt/C nanocomposite and DNA/RNA hybridization for the detection of COVID-19. Talanta 2023;124804.
7. Zhang K, Fan Z, Huang Y, Ding Y, Xie M. A strategy combining 3D-DNA Walker and CRISPR-Cas12a trans-cleavage activity applied to MXene based electrochemiluminescent sensor for SARS-CoV-2 RdRp gene detection. Talanta 2022;236:122868.
8. Wu T, Ge Y, Zhao K, Zhu X, Chen Y, Wu B, Zhu F, Zhu B, Cui L. A reverse-transcription recombinase-aided amplification assay for the rapid detection of N gene of severe acute respiratory syndrome coronavirus 2(SARS-CoV-2). Virology 2020:549:1–4.
9. Song M, Pang SY, Guo F, Wong MC, Hao J. Fluoride-free 2D niobium carbide MXenes as stable and biocompatible nanoplatforms for electrochemical biosensors with ultrahigh sensitivity. Advanced Science 2020;7(24):2001546.
10. Li J, Chang H, Zhang N, He Y, Zhang D, Liu B, Fang Y. Recent advances in enzyme inhibition based-electrochemical biosensors for pharmaceutical and environmental analysis. Talanta 2023;253:124092.
11. Soomro RA, Jawaid S, Zhang P, Han X, Hallam KR, Karakuș S, Kilislioğlu A, Xu B, Willander M. NiWO4-induced partial oxidation of MXene for photoelectrochemical detection of prostate-specific antigen. Sensors and Actuators B: Chemical 2021 Feb 1;328:129074.
12. Zaidi SA, Sheikh H, Al-Mahasna M, Elsin F. Crumpled MXene nanosheets for sensing of ascorbic acid in food, biological fluids, and erythrocytes in-vitro microenvironment. International Journal of Biological Macromolecules 2023 Sep 30;249:126024.
13. Xu B, Zhi C, Shi P. Latest Advances in MXene-based biosensors. J Phys: Mater 2020:3. https://doi.org/10.1088/2515-7639/ab8f78
14. Khan R, Andreescu S. Mxenes-based bioanalytical sensors: Design, characterization, and applications. Sensors 2020 Sep 22;20(18):5434.
15. Khazaei M, Ranjbar A, Arai M, Sasaki T, Yunoki S. Electronic properties and applications of MXenes: A theoretical review. Journal of Materials Chemistry 2017;5(10):2488–503.
16. Wu L, Lu X, Dhanjai, Wu Z-S, Dong Y, Wang X, Zheng S, Chen J. 2D transition metal carbide MXene as a robust biosensing platform for enzyme

immobilization and ultrasensitive detection of phenol. Biosensors and Bioelectronics 2018;107: 69–75.
17. Kong Y, Zhu Y, Song J, Liu Q, Song L, Fei X, Li X. A novel multimode biosensor for sensitive detection of AFB1 in food based on Mxenes nano enzymes. Food Chemistry 2023 Jun 17:136645.
18. Ghodrati M, Mir A, Farmani A. Proposing of SPR biosensor based on 2D Ti3C2T x MXene for uric acid detection immobilized by uricase enzyme. Journal of Computational Electronics 2023 Feb;22(1):560–9.
19. Wang F, Yang CH, Duan M, Tang Y, Zhu JF. TiO_2 nanoparticle modified organ-like Ti_3C_2 MXene nanocomposite encapsulating hemoglobin for a mediator-free biosensor with excellent performances. Biosensors and Bioelectronics 2015;74:1022–1028.
20. Gao R, Song Y, Gao Y, Yang X, Bao SJ. Stable hemoglobin-based biosensor based on coordination-assisted microfluidic technology for hydrogen peroxide determination. Sensors and Actuators Reports 2023;5:100146.
21. Nagarajan RD, Sundaramurthy A, Sundramoorthy AK. Synthesis and characterization of MXene (Ti_3C_2Tx)/Iron oxide composite for ultrasensitive electrochemical detection of hydrogen peroxide. Chemosphere 2022;286:131478.
22. Tong X, Jiang L, Ao Q, Lv X, Song Y, Tang J. Highly stable glucose oxidase polynanogel@ MXene/chitosan electrochemical biosensor based on a multi-stable interface structure for glucose detection. Biosensors and Bioelectronics 2023 Dec 23:115942.
23. Shi LM, Pan JX, Zhou B, Jiang X. A new bifunctional electrochemical sensor for hydrogen peroxide and nitrite based on a bimetallic metalloporphyrinic framework. Journal of Materials Chemistry B 2015;3(48):9340–9348.
24. Liu H, Duan C, Yang C, Shen W, Wang F, Zhu Z. A novel nitrite biosensor based on the direct electrochemistry of hemoglobin immobilized on MXene-Ti_3C_2. Sensors and Actuators B: Chemical 2015;218:60–66.
25. Wang Y, Zeng Z, Qiao J, Dong S, Liang Q, Shao S. Ultrasensitive determination of nitrite based on electrochemical platform of AuNPs deposited on PDDA-modified MXene nanosheets. Talanta 2021; 221:121605.
26. Wang T, Wang C, Xu X, Li Z, Li D. One-step electrodeposition synthesized Aunps/Mxene/ERGO for selectivity nitrite sensing. Nanomaterials (Basel) 2021 Jul 23;11(8):1892. https://doi.org/10.3390/nano11081892. PMID: 34443726; PMCID: PMC8401988.
27. Feng X, Han G, Cai J, Wang X. Au@Carbon quantum Dots-MXene nanocomposite as an electrochemical sensor for sensitive detection of nitrite. Journal of Colloid and Interface Science 2022 Feb;607(Pt 2):1313–1322. https://doi.org/10.1016/j.jcis.2021.09.036. Epub 2021 Sep 16. PMID: 34583036.
28. Pan, Y., He, M., Wu, J., Qi, H., Cheng, Y. One-Step synthesis of MXene-functionalized PEDOT: PSS conductive polymer hydrogels for wearable and noninvasive monitoring of sweat glucose. Sensors and Actuators B: Chemical 2023;135055.
29. Wu M, Zhang Q, Fang Y, Deng C, Zhou F, Zhang Y., ... Wang Y. Polylysine-modified MXene nanosheets with highly loaded glucose oxidase as cascade nanoreactor for glucose decomposition and electrochemical sensing. Journal of Colloid and Interface Science 2021;586:20–29.

30. Feng L, Qin W, Wang Y, Gu C, Li X, Chen J, Chen J, Qiao H, Yang M, Tian Z, Yin S. $Ti_3C_2T_x$ MXene/Graphene/AuNPs 3D porous composites for high sensitivity and fast response glucose biosensing. Microchem J 2023 Jan 1;184:108142.
31. Rakhi R, Nayak P, Xia C, et al. Novel amperometric glucose biosensor based on MXene nanocomposite. Scientific Reports 2016;6:36422. https://doi.org/10.1038/srep36422
32. Kumar S, Lei Y, Alshareef NH, Quevedo-Lopez MA, Salama KN. Biofunctionalized two-dimensional Ti_3C_2 MXenes for ultrasensitive detection of cancer biomarker. Biosensors and Bioelectronics 2018;121:243–249.
33. Song X, Gao H, Yuan R, Xiang Y. Trimetallic nanoparticle-decorated MXene nanosheets for catalytic electrochemical detection of carcinoembryonic antigen via Exo III-aided dual recycling amplifications. Sensors and Actuators B: Chemical 2022;359:131617.
34. Wu Q, Li N, Wang Y, Xu Y, Wei S, Wu J, ... Cui X. A 2D transition metal carbide MXene-based SPR biosensor for ultrasensitive carcinoembryonic antigen detection. Biosensors and Bioelectronics 2019;144:111697.
35. Luo W, Ye Z, Ma P, Wu Q, Song D. Preparation of a disposable electrochemiluminescence sensor chip based on an MXene-loaded ruthenium luminescent agent and its application in the detection of carcinoembryonic antigens. Analyst 2022;147(9):1986–94.
36. Kalkal A, Tiwari A, Sharma D, Baghel MK, Kumar P, Pradhan R, Packirisamy G. Air-brush spray coated Ti3C2-MXene-graphene nanohybrid thin film based electrochemical biosensor for cancer biomarker detection. International Journal of Biological Macromolecules 2023 Dec 31;253:127260.
37. Kumar D. Electrochemical immunosensor based on titanium dioxide grafted MXene for EpCAM antigen detection. Journal of Colloid and Interface Science 2023 Dec 15;652:549–56.
38. Khan R, Ben Aissa S, Sherazi TA, Catanante G, Hayat A, Marty JL. Development of an impedimetric aptasensor for label free detection of patulin in apple juice. Molecules 2019 Mar 13;24(6):1017.
39. Zheng J, Wang B, Ding A, Weng B, Chen J. Synthesis of MXene/DNA/Pd/Pt nanocomposite for sensitive detection of dopamine. Journal of Electroanalytical Chemistry 2018 May 1;816:189–94.
40. Yang X, Feng M, Xia J, Zhang F, Wang Z. An electrochemical biosensor based on AuNPs/Ti3C2 MXene three-dimensional nanocomposite for microRNA-155 detection by exonuclease III-aided cascade target recycling. Journal of Electroanalytical Chemistry 2020 Dec 1;878:114669.
41. Fan P, Ma E, Liu C, Zhao Y, Wen X, Wang L, Li L, Qu Q. A new electrochemical DNA biosensor based on the density control strategy of Ti3C2NH2 MXene@Au nanocomposites for the detection of hepatitis B virus-DNA. Ionics 2023 Oct 31:1–2.
42. Zhang J, Li Y, Duan S, He F. Highly electrically conductive two-dimensional Ti3C2 Mxenes-based 16S rDNA electrochemical sensor for detecting Mycobacterium tuberculosis. Analytica Chimica Acta. 2020 Aug 1;1123:9–17.
43. Wang L, Cui K, Wang P, Pei M, Guo W. A sensitive electrochemical DNA sensor for detecting *Helicobacter pylori* based on accordion-like Ti3C2Tx: A simple strategy. Analytical and Bioanalytical Chemistry. 2021 Jul;413:4353–62.

3

MXene-Based Emerging 2D Materials for Biomarkers (Electrodes)

Lizaranee Tripathy, Ashish K. Sarangi, Rajiv Lochan Bal, Puneet K. Singh, Snehasish Mishra, Ajit Behera, and Ranjan K. Mohapatra

3.1 Introduction

MXenes are newly created two-dimensional (2D) materials resembling graphene in structure and characteristics. MXene is a class of carbide, nitride, or carbonitride of (2D) transition metal regarded as the most promising candidate for biomedical applications due to its exceptional aspect range, atomic-thin thickness, maximum dispersal power in an aqueous system, minimal cytotoxicity, and flawless photothermal performance [1]. MXenes, pronounced 'maxenes,' are currently the fastest-growing family of 2D materials [2]. The elements used to build MXenes, MAX phases and their intercalated ions, are shown in Figure 3.1. Numerous applications of these compounds have been reported to date. A pie chart showing the annual publications (applications and properties) of MXenes from 2011 to 2019 is shown in Figure 3.2.

Biomarkers are indicators used to monitor and regulate biological functions and human health. They are a tool to analyze physiological traits like blood pressure, cholesterol level, and urine to detect and pre-empt health status. They can also recommend appropriate intervention measures. The National Institutes of Health (NIH; in the US) states that a biological molecule found in tissues, blood, or other bodily fluids is called a biomarker, indicating a disease condition or process aberration [3]. The concentration and activity of biomarkers in a biological setting can be measured to forecast the progression of a disease or offer relevant data to decide on treatment prescriptions [4]. As a result, big businesses and domain experts are interested in applying biomarker-based analytical techniques [5]. Many recent applied research findings on using analytical methods to quantify biomarkers to assess and regulate bodily activity in sports and medical studies have been reported [6]. Biosensors enjoy plenty of attention as possible alternatives to intricate, costly,

DOI: 10.1201/9781003353287-3

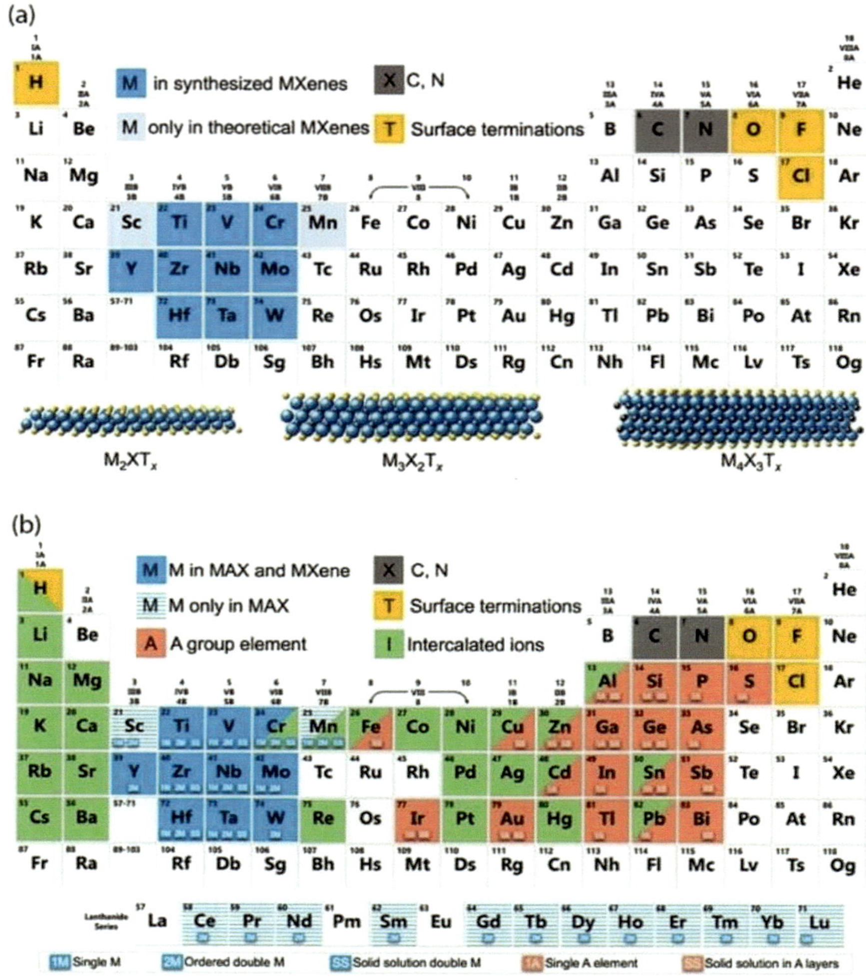

FIGURE 3.1
Representation showing compositions of MXenes and MAX phases in Periodic table. (a) Elements used to build MXenes, (b) elements used to build MAX phases, MXenes, and their intercalated ions [2].

and spacious conventional analytical procedures as conventionally employed in medical sciences [7]. Currently, major areas in biosensor research include the rapid and precise detection of biochemicals or biomolecules responsible for chronic disease and adverse health effects to enable early enhanced diagnosis and timely therapeutic interventions [7,8]. Due to their biocompatibility and suitability in detecting biological molecules, an array of nanomaterials (like carbon nanotubes and transition metal dichalcogenides) has lately been

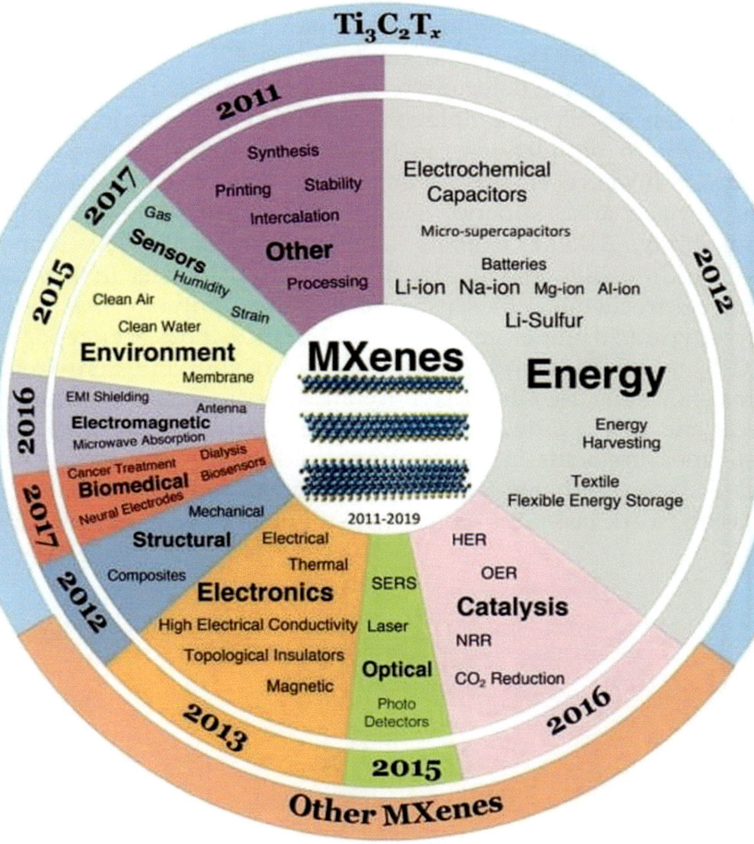

FIGURE 3.2
A pie chart showing the annual publications (applications and properties) of MXenes from 2011 to 2019 [2].

employed in developing electrochemical sensor-based biosensors [9,10]. Owing to their distinct surface chemicals' properties like hydrophilicity, a wide range of varying compositions, an abundance of MXenes have many uses in the development of electrochemical biosensors due to their surface functional groups, biocompatibility, exceptional electrocatalytic activity, strong electron transfer ability, and ease of surface functionalization and modification, among the many 2D-layered nanomaterials [11]. There has not been much progress made in the field of continuous health monitoring [12]. This is due to numerous unresolved issues, including low analyte concentrations for sensing response collection, biofouling, biocompatibility, and smaller biofluid ampoule quantity [13,14]. Like carbides, nitrides, and carbonitrides, MXene is primarily classified as an early transition metal. Like graphene, it is regarded as a wonder material due to its immense potential for a variety of uses, including in energy storage and conversion [15], use as electrochemical sensors [16], and in catalysis [17].

Further, as most of the detectors need blood samples due to the invasive nature of biosensors, blood sample collection from the geriatric, hemophobic, and the newborn populations can be challenging [18]. Wearable electrochemical non-invasive biosensors are still being perfected. Because of its superior surface area, superior electrical characteristics, and improved biocompatibility, MXene exhibits a remarkable ability to immobilize enzymes. Additionally, it facilitates direct electron transfer in enzymes. To create an electrochemical biosensor for β-hydroxybutyrate that detects β-hydroxybutyric acid amperometrically, for instance, it has been reported [19] that $Ti_3C_2T_x$ nanosheets were coated with β-hydroxybutyrate dehydrogenase. A schema shows the use β-hydroxybutyrate dehydrogenase to create MXene 2D sheets and detect β-hydroxybutyric acid. Currently, handling accurate biosensor measurements in practical applications through biosensor technologies is laden with numerous operational circumstance-related issues (i.e., mission/work task conditions) that still need to be resolved. Although

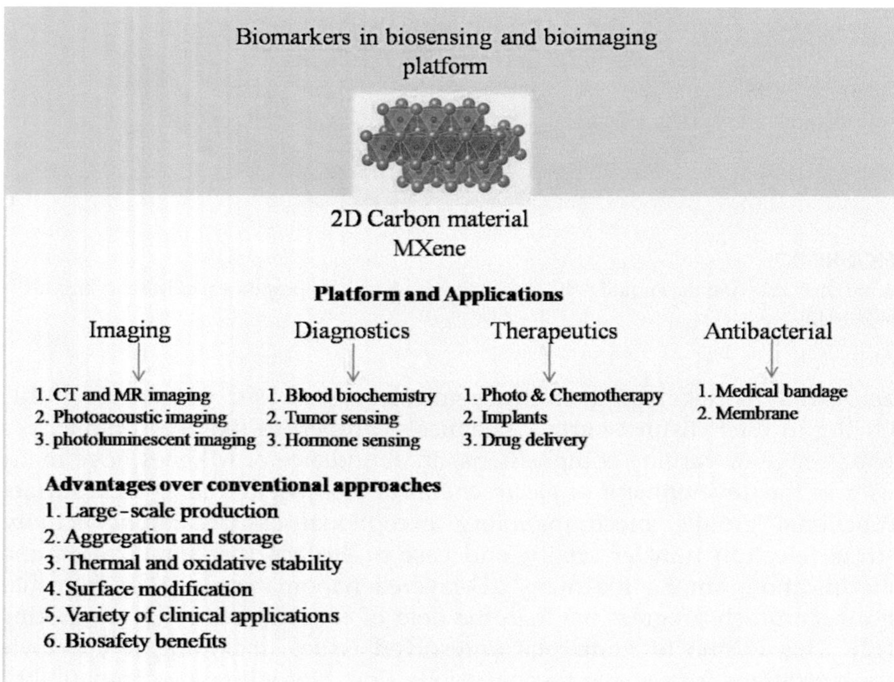

FIGURE 3.3
Common technologies using biomarkers in the detection and sensing platforms.

the health-relevant biomarker sensors have been reviewed a number of times [20], the majority of them have described these only in laboratory settings. This chapter's originality lies in its description of HHPM-specific sensor technologies emphasizing the psychophysiological biomarkers while discussing how to detect these biomarkers in a variety of settings, hence addressing real-world challenges [21]. While it covers the extensively prevalent and widely utilized technology linked to the identification of biomarkers and sensing platforms (Figure 3.3), it was impossible to include them all due to space limitations.

3.2 MXene-Based Electrodes as Biomarkers

This section discusses using MXene material-incorporated electrochemical (bio)sensors to recognize drugs, environmental pollutants, and health- and wellbeing-related biomarkers, with a brief background of the sensor, its fabrication, and the underlying electrochemical reaction when applied. The objective is to highlight the improved electrochemical strengths and qualities (LOD, stability, sensitivity, detection range, etc.), and additionally the shortcomings of the sensor [22]. The architecture, large surface area, and biodegradability and hydrophilicity are among the most alluring characteristics of MXenes in electrochemical sensing; these can be combined to modify the electrode surfaces with additional nanomaterials and sensing characteristics. Conventional detection techniques like mass spectrometry, chromatography, and immunoassay involve labor-intensive sample preparation, expensive analysis procedures, and elaborate infrastructure, all of which are relatively demanding.

In contrast to this, nanomaterial-based electrochemical (bio)sensors can rapidly detect, are highly sensitive and selective, and have simple designs [23–28]. Zhang et al. [29] created an electrochemical sensor for simultaneous detection of acetaminophen (ACOP) and isoniazid (INZ) using Ti_3C_2Tx MXene, enabling high sensitivity, low reagent usage, and low-cost medical diagnosis and monitoring. They described MXene/DNA/Pd/Pt electrochemical sensors to measure dopamine [30], where MXene serves as a conductive matrix to Pd/Pt nanoparticle loading; the aromatic hydrophobic base adsorbs DNA on the MXene sheet surface that encourages Pd/Pt nanoparticle formation in vivo. The sensor was developed by covering a glassy carbon electrode with MXene/DNA/Pd/Pt slurry immobilized using Nafion solution. A MXene/DNA/Pd/Pt sensor demonstrated amplified amperometric response to dopamine at 0.2–1000 μM, with a 30 nM detection limit. Dopamine detection sensitivity was possible due to the harmonious working of electrode components. The sensor electrode also had a significant dopamine selectivity, which is essential for sensitive detection. The sensor was incredibly dopamine selective when molecules like glucose, AA, and UA were present with oxidation potentials close to dopamine. Without a matrix effect, the sensor could identify dopamine in human serum samples.

3.2.1 Detecting Oncogenesis

Cancer is a serious threat to human life and it is medically challenging to ensure well-being of patients. As per the American Cancer Society estimates, the US recorded 1,762,450 new cancer cases in 2019, and cancer-related fatalities are expected to increase to 606,880 soon. About 4,829 are diagnosed with cancer, and roughly 1,663 individuals die of cancer, every day in the US. Cancer incidence and death can be substantially reduced through early diagnosis and effective treatment. Apart from elevated rates of morbidity and mortality, an additional grave cancer-associated concern is the exacerbated socioeconomic disparity wherein avoidable cancer causes a significant financial disparity. The mortality in lung and liver cancers in males was 40% higher and cervical cancer mortality was two times higher in the developing world than in the developed nations between 2012 and 2016 [31,32]. It is critical to create low-cost, non-invasive techniques for cancer theranostics. An intricate clinical setting is needed to diagnose oncogenic tumors, including X-ray, CT, MRI, biopsy, cytology, endoscopy, sonography, positron emission tomography (PET), and thermography. Growing popular techniques like immunohistochemistry (IHC), radioimmunoassay (RIA), polymerase chain reaction (PCR), enzyme-linked immunosorbent test (ELISA), and flow cytometry use genomic and proteomic (molecular) tools. However, most of the currently employed techniques and procedures are time-consuming, costly, intrusive, and have suitable laboratory set-up only in larger hospitals. Biosensors are a great substitute for intricate instrumentation facilities with the ability to offer prompt, precise, and sensitive early identification; track cancer spread and angiogenesis; and test non-invasively to evaluate the efficacy of anticancer chemotherapy. Electrochemical biosensors are advantageous due to their low cost, simplicity, ease of miniaturization, and mass fabrication. They serve as point-of-care resources, with gadgets able to be set-up in locations such as a doctor's office or at home. Thus, they have gained much interest and much work has gone into creating highly selective and ultrasensitive electrochemical biosensors to detect cancer markers [33]. Developing novel redox tags for radiometric electrochemical and multiplex assays, creating nanomaterial-based signal amplifiers, integrating electrochemical biosensors with microfluidic chips, and designing high specificity and affinity receptors are some of the efforts that have been made. Figure 3.4A presents the benefits, constituent elements, and diverse electrochemical assessment techniques. Uncontrolled cell proliferation is typically a cause of cancers accomplished by numerous cellular events such as tumor formation, migrating cancer cells, tumor metastasis, and specific genomic alterations that precede transcriptome and protein alteration. Malignant cells typically exhibit altered phenotype, metabolism, and size compared to normal cells. Alterations occur in the tumor-associated microenvironment [34]. When immune cells come into contact with cancer cells, they release specific cytokines [35,36]. The matrix metalloproteinases also cause dramatic extracellular matrix alterations. Numerous distinct cancer biomarkers, including altered genomics, microRNA, cytokines, MMPs, exosomes, cancer antigens, circulating tumor DNA (ctDNA), and circulating tumor cells are created during tumorigenesis and its progression to metastasis. Figure 3.4B presents cancer biomarkers at the source, during migration, and colonization at a secondary site.

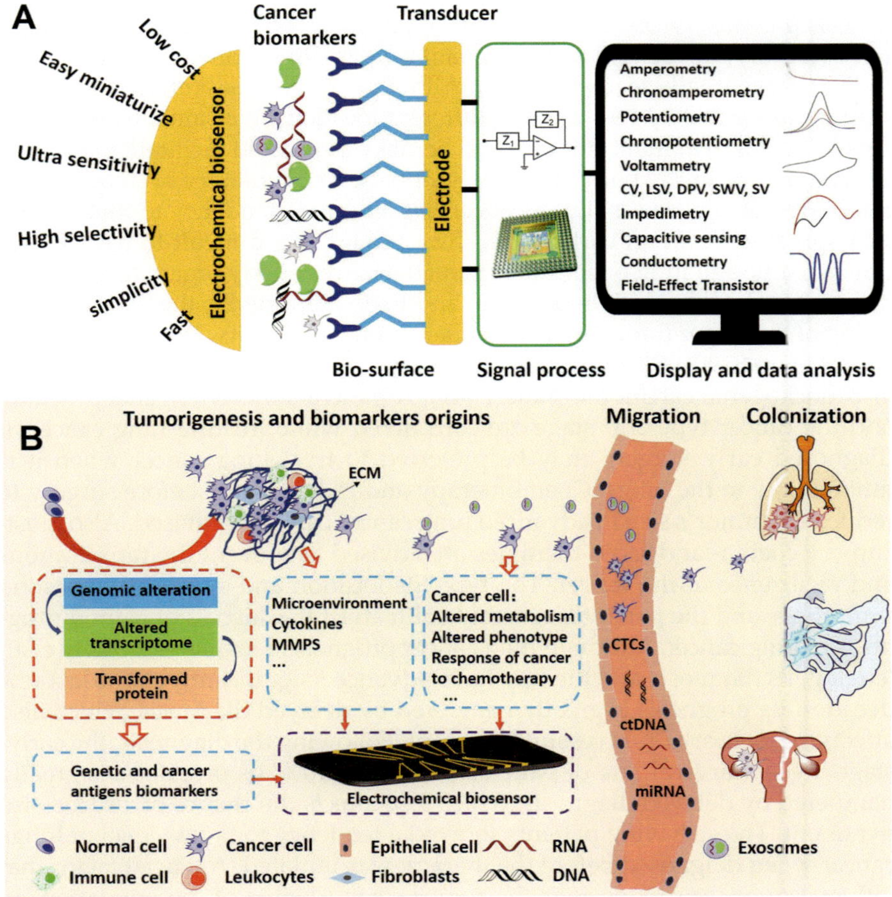

FIGURE 3.4

(A) The benefits, constituent elements, and diverse electrochemical assessment techniques; (B) the biomarkers that originate from cancer, its migration, and colonization to a secondary site [34].

3.2.1.1 Detecting Lung Cancer

Cancer is a common illness impacting more than 60 human organs and is presented in more than 200 forms [37]. The initial phase of the spread of oncotumors accounts for almost 90% of all cancer-related fatalities [38]. Lung cancer affects more than 1.76 million people globally, accounting for approximately 25% of all cancer-related fatalities, and is a cancer that has a severe impact on health and well-being [39]. Molecular, genetic, and epigenetic level anomalies, like any other malignancy, cause lung cancer.

The human body typically has a check-and-balance mechanism to regulate the growth and division of cells, and new cells are produced only when necessary. The complete sequence of the cellular process for this is referred to as apoptosis, or programmed cell death. When apoptosis fails and tumorigenesis prevails, unchecked cell division produces a benign or malignant cell mass (tumor) [40]. Benign and malignant tumors differ from each other, where the latter eventually leads to cancer. Although surgery is preferred to treat a benign tumor to stop its spread to different locations, the same invasive process to treat a malignant tumor could be risky as it could facilitate the spread of malignancy in the body through lymphatic or circulatory systems; this is referred to as metastasis. Lung cancer has an innate tendency to metastasize and spread even at an early stage, thus making it a difficult-to-treat severe illness. Although lung oncotumors can attack every body organ, they usually target the adrenal gland, liver, brain, and bone. Reportedly, the epithelial cell lining of the larger (bronchi) and smaller (bronchioles) airways is the primary source of up to 90–95% lung malignancy. Thus, lung malignancy is also known as bronchogenic carcinoma/cancer [41]. A patient's lifestyle, general health, and the cancer type and stage are considered while treating lung cancer. If diagnosed early, surgery may be preferred to treat lung cancer when it is limited only to the lungs. Chemotherapy and radiotherapy before surgery to reduce the tumor's size in advanced lung cancer cases are advised. Also, post-surgery chemo- and radio-therapies are advised to prevent the ramifications and recurrence of the cancer. The type, its location and spread, the existing symptoms, and the patient's general health affect the success of a good prognosis of lung cancer. Although lung cancer prognosis remains extremely challenging, its diagnosis and therapy have advanced significantly in the last few decades. Its prognosis is greatly hampered by delayed diagnosis, which also affects the chance of a successful treatment. Following the diagnosis, the early-stage 5-year survival rate of patients is about 5–10%. Its prognosis is greatly hampered by delayed diagnosis, which also affects the chance of a successful treatment. The surviving patients showed a tendency for a low level of lungs cancer when diagnosed before the therapy was initiated. A crucial factor that influences cancer prognosis is the tumor stage (degree of dissemination) in non-small cell lung cancer (NSCLC) during diagnosis. Surgery can eliminate stage I tumors, with a 5-year survival rate close to 75% [42]. Thus, sensitive and reliable lung cancer prognosis and diagnosis instruments are necessary.

3.2.1.2 Detecting Pancreatic Cancer

The fourth most common cause of cancer-related deaths in the US is pancreatic cancer. An estimated 43,140 new pancreatic cancer cases are likely to be reported annually, with an astounding 36,800 lives lost. While the pancreas can develop a wide range of malignancies, most (85–90%) of these tumors are pancreatic ductal adenocarcinomas, a particular histological subtype. A dismal prognosis and an inability to detect the cancer early while there is still hope for curative resection are the primary causes of this high fatality rate. The deep, inaccessible position of the pancreas in the belly, the early growth of metastases, and the late presentation of symptoms like weight loss, epigastric pain, or obstructive jaundice, are some factors contributing to this challenge. As a result, most pancreatic cancer patients have incurable illness at diagnosis, resulting in a 6-month median survival and an overall <5% 5-year survival rate [43]. Contrarily, recovery can reach 20–30% for 5-year survival for the few individuals who arrive with tiny, surgically resectable tumors [44]. However, mass screening of the general population may not be cost-effective and is thus not suggested [45]. Efforts may be focused on the early screening of symptomatic outpatients, with a 79% (70–90%) median sensitivity (SN) and 82% (68–91%) median specificity (SP). However, it is demonstrably unsuccessful while screening many asymptomatic cases.

3.2.1.3 Detecting Breast Cancer

Biomarkers are essential to manage breast cancer, particularly when selecting a systemic medication. The European Group of Tumor Markers (EGTM) issued recommendations for using biomarkers in breast cancer for the first time in 2005 [46]. Significant advancements, particularly in tissue-based biomarkers, have been documented since then. This includes using HER2 to determine the likelihood of an early response to various anti-HER2 therapies and using multi-parameter signatures to predict prognosis. Thus, updated guidelines to conduct biomarker tests for breast cancer, like HER2, progesterone receptors, and estrogen receptors, have been released. To update the guidelines, literature available online at PubMed and Cochrane library on the application of breast cancer biomarkers during June 2005 and June 2016 was examined, which was similar to earlier announcements of the guidelines [47].

The target audiences for these guidelines are medical professionals like physicians, surgeons, and nurses treating breast cancer patients, and lab experts working on cancer biomarkers. The suggestions made under the guidelines may also help medical professionals, health policy decision-makers, breast cancer researchers, regulatory bodies, afflicted individuals, and businesses producing or distributing targeted diagnostics and therapeutics.

3.2.1.4 Detecting Ovarian Cancer

One type of gynecological cancer is ovarian cancer, ranking second in terms of the number of global deaths, accounting for about 151,000 annually, owing to delayed detection. Notwithstanding advancements in its treatment over the past few decades, the rate of survival has only marginally increased. Ovarian cancer is multifaceted and includes both epithelial and non-epithelial types and subtypes identified through combined anatomical and clinical factors [48]. A widely used serum biomarker to detect ovarian cancer is cancer antigen-125 (CA125) [13], originally identified and reported by an American scientist in 1981 [49,50]. The MUC16 gene encodes CA125, commonly known as Mucin 16 (MUC16), a high molecular weight (>200 kDa) glycoprotein. Released either in soluble body fluid form or expressed as a membrane-bound protein on the cell surface, it undergoes meta-plastic differentiation into the epithelium of the Mullerian type CA125, a crucial tumor biomarker produced by ovarian epithelial cell and mesothelial cell tumors whose focus within the body fluid correlates with specific physical parameters.

Biosensors have become a significant cutting-edge tool in diagnostics over the last few decades, and their usage is expanding quickly, particularly at point-of-care diagnostics. High CA125 detection and quantification approaches that are both sensitive and selective have been published using distinct identification elements and sensing concepts and techniques. These provide a synopsis of electrochemical, piezoelectric, and optical biosensing techniques, such as chemiluminescence, fluorescence resonance energy transfer-electrochemical biosensing, field-effect transistor-based electrochemical biosensing, potentiometric-based electrochemical biosensing, focused surface plasmon resonance-based optical biosensing, amperometric-based electrochemical biosensing, and impedimetric-based electrochemical biosensing [49–62].

3.2.1.5 Detecting Colorectal Cancer

Colorectal cancer claims more than 500,000 lives annually globally, affecting millions of men and women [63]. Colorectal cancer was ranked third among malignant cancers in Europe in both men and women in 2010 [64]. A total of 250,000 colorectal cancer cases are diagnosed each year in Europe alone. The 5-year survival rate for 1995–1999 for adult Europeans diagnosed with colorectal cancer was 54% [65]. According to recent studies, the overall relative 5-year survival can reach 65%, although this may vary depending on the cancer stage [3]. Biomarkers-based testing continues to increase.

In most cases, DNA, RNA, microRNA (miRNA), epigenetic modifications, or antibodies are included in defining a biomarker. There are many proteins or glycolipids that are part of the biological structures of normal cells during the various stages of cell development which are usually termed as 'biomarkers.'

However, a few of these biomarkers can actively participate as the cell develops carcinogenesis which the oncologists consider as 'tumor markers.' Thus every tumor marker is a biomarker, while the reverse may not be true. . Tumor-associated antigens, which comprise the largest group of clinically important indicators, are an example of such a material. Because of this, the focus of tumor-associated antigens usually correlates with the mass (number) of particular neoplastic cells. Numerous sensitive, specific, and predictive well-established value measures are employed in clinical practices during diagnosis and therapy. Research indicates that some factors are more crucial for long-term follow-up and treatment. These chemicals produced by cells were considered in observational research, clinical trials, and long-term lab tests. Tumor markers quantified in diagnosis can be used during screening to help detect cancer early. For some tumor forms, markers are crucial to track the efficiency of chemotherapy, radiotherapy, surgery, neo-adjuvant therapy, and follow-up to ensure that the cancer does not recur. Extended observational research indicates that tracking the development and dynamics of an antigen can be as crucial as estimating its content [66].

3.2.2 Detecting Blood Biomarkers (Uric Acid, Creatinine, and Urea)

As per a survey, about 17 Indians out of every 100 have chronic kidney disease. Renal disease at its third stage, wherein immediate dialysis or kidney transplant is necessitated, is estimated to affect 6% of Indians [67–69]. About 30–60% of renal impairments are linked to diabetes and hypertension, and India is reportedly the second most diabetic country in the world. Kidney transplantation is not opted for by many due to the high expense. Renal problems may be diagnosed when acute. Further, discrepancies in the typical ranges of particular physiological parameters found in human bodily fluids might be utilized as biomarkers to identify kidney diseases by acting as signs of aberrant renal function [70,71]. The responses of biomarkers during diagnostic and therapeutic interventions have been studied. Research on how the biomarkers respond to therapeutic and diagnostic interventions has also been carried out (Figure 3.5). Although a biomarker is produced in an unusually large quantity during illness, the degree of aberrant renal biomarkers content finally serves as a determining factor. The likelihood of renal malfunction is determined by factors such as preeclampsia, diabetic nephropathy, kidney malignancy, and improper glomerular filtration rate [72].

Research on renal biomarkers in different bodily fluids (such as sweat, tears, urine, plasma, etc.) to detect acute kidney disease/disorder and prevent disease severity by providing prompt and efficient treatment is being carried out. Quality biomarkers to diagnose kidney illnesses may have the following qualifying features:

a. They ought to be affordable, simple to use, rapid in response, and unintrusive; blood and urine are readily accessible good biomarker sources for renal diagnosis.

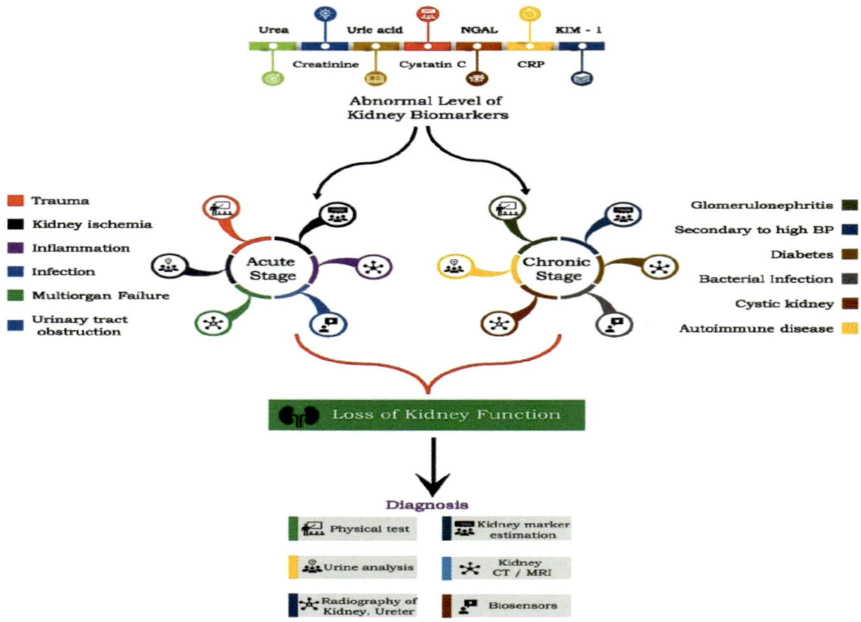

FIGURE 3.5
An illustration of the numerous renal function biomarkers, numerous chronic and acute disorders linked to distinct kidney biomarkers, and the various biomarker-based techniques used in testing and identifying kidney function loss [72].

b. They must have high sensitivity to differentiate the concentrations between the samples of ill and healthy individuals.
c. They need to be precise and should produce rapid and accurate analytical signals while diagnosing a renal illness.
d. Biomarkers need to make sense of physiological events, and provide sufficient information to comprehend how they are related.

Nitrogenous compounds in the human body other than proteins, like amino acids, uric acid, and creatinine, are called nonprotein nitrogen. Among these, creatinine and uric acid are necessary metabolites of proteins and nucleic acids. The human body usually produces and distributes endogenous and exogenous creatinine and uric acid, which are removed via glomerular filtration. The body produces uric acid, a highly soluble urate, as a purine metabolism byproduct [73]. The blood and urine uric acid levels in healthy humans, respectively, range between 240–520 μM and 1.44–4.43mM on average [74]. Altered uric acid levels indicate a disorder. Dramatic changes in the human diet and eating more purine-rich food with increased living standards have increased the risk of hyperuricemia and gout. Investigations essentially also link high uric acid levels to hypertension and fatty liver [75].

3.2.3 Detecting Biochemical Analytes in Blood Serum

Samples of blood or serum are expected to be loaded sources of prostate cancer (PCa) biomarkers. Human Kallikrein-3 PSA remains the most favored and first option approach as the gold standard for diagnosis and detection. The US FDA (Food and Drug Administration) vouched for PSA and DRE for prostate cancer identification and diagnosis in 1994. A blood PSA value of <4 ng/mL in an individual is the cut-off for prostate cancer confirmation. Some positive cases are reported at between 4 and 10 ng/mL. It is noteworthy that benign prostatic hyperplasia (BPH), prostate inflammation, and a PSA result of more than 4.0 ng/mL are correlated [76]. Experience over the previous 20 years hints at the lack of specificity in PSA-based detection as its primary drawback; biopsy reports confirmed a negative result even when the PSA level was between 4.0 and 10.0 ng/mL in about 75% of cases [77]. Prostate cancer patients with a PSA level of ~2.0 ng/mL in the previous year before diagnosis reportedly had a greater chance of fatality following radical prostatectomy. Analyzing the widely used PSA biomarkers could help in overcoming the drawbacks of prostate biopsy and enhance evaluation precision [78]. Thus, prostate cancer symptoms cannot be diagnosed using PSA-based techniques alone.

3.3 Conclusion

From the above discussion, using MXene-based electrodes for biomarker detection is a promising avenue in biosensing and medical diagnostics. The diverse applications explored here highlight the versatility and potential impact of MXene-based electrodes in detecting various cancers like liver, colorectal, ovarian, lung, pancreatic, and breast to identifying blood biomarkers such as uric acid, creatinine, and urea, and the analysis of biochemical analytes in blood sera. High conductivity, large surface area, and excellent biocompatibility are some of the unique properties of MXenes that contribute to their efficacy as sensing platforms. These qualities improve the selectivity and sensitivity of detecting a biomarker, and addressing critical challenges in early disease diagnosis and monitoring. This chapter has discussed and underscored the progress in leveraging MXene materials to develop efficient and reliable biosensors for various clinical applications.

However, just like any new technology, there are challenges and shortcomings to resolve. These include optimizing the stability and reproducibility of MXene-based electrodes, standardizing the fabrication techniques, and ensuring scalability for practical implementation. MXene-based electrodes hold great promise in advancing the field of biomarker detection, offering a platform that can revolutionize medical diagnostics while contributing to the evolving personalized and precision medicines. Continued interdisciplinary research and collaboration between material scientists, biologists, and clinicians is essential to overcoming these challenges and unlocking the full potential of MXene-based electrodes in clinical settings. It is anticipated that MXene-based biosensors will play a pivotal role in enhancing the ability to detect diseases early, monitor the treatment responses, and ultimately improve patient outcomes in health care with the progress in cutting-edge research and breakthrough discoveries.

References

1. Chaturvedi, K., Hada, V., Paul, S., Sarma, B., Malvi, D., Dhangar, M., Bajpai, H., Singhwane, A., Srivastava, A.K., Verma, S. (2023). The rise of MXene: A wonder 2D material, from its synthesis and properties to its versatile applications—A comprehensive review. Topics in Current Chemistry, 381(2), 11.
2. Gogotsi, Y., Anasori, B. (2019). The rise of MXenes. American Chemical Society Nano, 13, 8491–8494.
3. Langan, R.C., Mullinax, J.E., Raiji, M.T., Upham, T., Summers, T., Stojadinovic, A., Avital, I. (2013). Colorectal cancer biomarkers and the potential role of cancer stem cells. Journal of Cancer, 4, 241–250.
4. Argiriadis, E., Martino, M., Segnana, M., Poto, L., Vecchiato, M., Battistel, D., Gambaro, A., Barbante, C. (2020). Multi-proxy biomarker determination in peat: Optimized extraction and cleanup method for paleoenvironmental application. Microchemical Journal, 156 (July 2020), 104821.
5. Yoshinobu, T., Ecken, H., Poghossian, A., Lüth, H., Iwasaki, H., Schoning, M.J. (2001). Alternative sensor materials for light-addressable potentiometric sensors. Sensors and Actuators B: Chemical, 76 (1–3), 388–392.
6. Orooji, Y., Sohrabi, H., Hemmat, N., Oroojalian, F., Baradaran, B., Mokhtarzadeh, A., Mohaghegh, M., Karimi-Maleh, H. (2020). An overview on SARS-CoV-2 (COVID-19) and other human coronaviruses and their detection capability via amplification assay, chemical sensing, biosensing, immunosensing, and clinical assays. Nano-Micro Letters, 13 (1), 1–30.
7. Kirsch, J., Siltanen, C., Zhou, Q., Revzin, A., Simonian, A. (2013). Biosensor technology: recent advances in threat agent detection and medicine. Chemical Society Reviews, 42, 8733–8768, https://doi.org/10.1039/C3CS60141B.
8. Park, Y.M., Ahn, J., Choi, Y.S., Jeong, J.-M., Lee, S.J., Lee, J.J., Choi, B.G., Lee, K.G. (2020). Flexible nanopillar-based immunoelectrochemical biosensor for noninvasive detection of Amyloid beta. Nano Convergence, 7, 29.
9. Hussein, M.A., El-Said, W.A., Abu-Zied, B.M., Choi, J.-W. (2020). Nanosheet composed of gold nanoparticle/graphene/epoxy resin based on ultrasonic fabrication for flexible dopamine biosensor using surface-enhanced Raman spectroscopy. Nano Convergence, 7, 15, https://doi.org/10.1186/s40580-020-00225-8.

10. Wee, Y., Park, S., Kwon, Y.H., Ju, Y., Yeon, K.-M., Kim, J. (2019). Tyrosinaseimmobilized CNT based biosensor for highly-sensitive detection of phenolic compounds. Biosensors and Bioelectronics, 132, 279–285.
11. Yoon, J., Shin, M., Lim, J., Lee, J.-Y., Choi, J.-W. (2020). Recent advances in MXene nanocomposite-based biosensors. Biosensors, 10, 185.
12. Windmiller, J.R., Wang, J. (2013). Wearable electrochemical sensors and biosensors: A review. Electroanalysis, 25, 29–46.
13. Song, H.-J., Yim, J.-K., Park, C.-Y., Kim, Y.-S., Kim, J.-D. (2013). Comparison of the diagnostic performances of CA125 and multiple marker combinations for early diagnosis of ovarian cancer. International Journal of Bio-Science and Bio-Technology, 5, 141–150.
14. Hammock, M.L., Chortos, A., Tee, B.C.-K., Tok, J.B.-H., Bao, Z. (2013). 25th anniversary article: The evolution of electronic skin (E-Skin): a brief history, design considerations, and recent progress. Advanced Materials, 25, 5997–6038.
15. Verma, S., Dwivedi, U., Chaturvedi, K., Kumari, N., Dhangar, M., Hashmi, S.A., Singhal, R., Srivastava, A.K. (2022). Progress of 2D MXenes based composites for efficient electromagnetic interference shielding applications: A review. Synthetic Metals, 287, 117095.
16. Das, P., Wu, Z.-S. (2020). MXene for energy storage: Present status and future perspectives. Journal of Physics: Energy, 2, 032004, https://doi.org/10.1088/2515-7655/ab9b1d.
17. Kalambate, P.K., Gadhari, N.S., Li, X., Rao, Z., Navale, S.T., Shen, Y., Patil, V.R., Huang, Y. (2019). Recent advances in MXene–based electrochemical sensors and biosensors. TrAC Trends in Analytical Chemistry, 120, 115643.
18. Bandodkar, A.J., Wang, J. (2014). Non-invasive wearable electrochemical sensors: A review. Trends in Biotechnology, 32, 363–371, https://doi.org/10.1016/j.tibtech.2014.04.005.
19. Koyappayil, A., Chavan, S.G., Mohammadniaei, M., Go, A., Hwang, S.Y., Lee, M.-H. (2020). b-Hydroxybutyrate dehydrogenase decorated MXene nanosheets for the amperometric determination of b-hydroxybutyrate. Microchimica Acta, 187, 277.
20. Heikenfeld, J., Jajack, A., Rogers, J., Gutruf, P., Tian, L., Pan, T., Li, R., Khine, M., Kim, J., Wang, J., Kim, J. (2018). Wearable sensors: Modalities, challenges, and prospects. Lab on a Chip, 18, 217.
21. Jayathilaka, W.A.D.M., Qi, K., Qin, Y., Chinnappan, A., Serrano- Garcia, W., Baskar, C., Wang, H., He, J., Cui, S., Thomas, S.W., Ramakrishna, S. (2019). Significance of nanomaterials in wearables: A review on wearable actuators and sensors. Advanced Materials, 31, 1805921.
22. Wang, F., Yang, C.H., Duan, C.Y., Xiao, D., Tang, Y., Zhu, J.F. (2015). An organelike titanium carbide material (MXene) with multilayer structure encapsulating hemoglobin for a mediatorfree biosensor, Journal of the Electrochemical Society, 162, B16eB21.
23. Kalambate, P.K., Sanghavi, B.J., Karna, S.P., Srivastava, A.K. (2015). Simultaneous voltammetric determination of paracetamol and domperidone based on a graphene/platinum nanoparticles/nafion composite modified glassy carbon electrode. Sensors and Actuators B: Chemical, 213, 285–294.
24. Kalambate, P.K., Srivastava, A.K. (2016). Simultaneous voltammetric determination of paracetamol, cetirizine and phenylephrine using a multiwalled

carbon nanotubeeplatinum nanoparticles nanocomposite modified carbon paste electrode, Sensors and Actuators B: Chemical, 233, 237–248.
25. Kalambate, P.K., Rawool, C.R., Srivastava, A.K. (2016). Voltammetric determination of pyrazinamide at grapheneezinc oxide nanocomposite modified carbon paste electrode employing differential pulse voltammetry. Sensors and Actuators B: Chemical, 237, 196–205.
26. Kalambate, P.K., Dhanjai, Huang, Z., Li, Y., Shen, Y., Xie, M., Huang, Y., Srivastava, A.K. (2019). Core@Shell nanomaterials based sensing devices: A review. Trends in Analytical Chemistry, 115, 147–161.
27. Singhwane, A., Chaturvedi, K., Mohapatra, R.K., Srivastava, A.K., Verma, S. (2023). Mxene-based composite materials as antibacterial agents for healthcare applications (Chapter 1). ACS Symposium Series, 1443, 1–17, https://doi.org/10.1021/bk-2023-1443.ch001.
28. Sinha, A., Dhanjai, Tan, B., Huang, Y., Zhao, H., Dang, X., Chen, J., Jain, R. (2018). MoS2 nanostructures for electrochemical sensing of multidisciplinary targets: A review. Trends in Analytical Chemistry, 102, 75e90.
29. Zhang, Y., Jiang, X., Zhang, J., Zhang, H., Li, Y. (2019). Simultaneous voltammetric determination of acetaminophen and isoniazid using MXene modified screen-printed electrode. Biosensors and Bioelectronics, 130, 315–321.
30. Zheng, J., Wang, B., Ding, A., Weng, B., Chen, J. (2018). Synthesis of MXene/DNA/Pd/Pt nanocomposite for sensitive detection of dopamine. Journal of Electroanalytical Chemistry, 816, 189–194.
31. Prabhakar, B., Shende, P., Augustine, S. (2018). Current trends and emerging diagnostic techniques for lung cancer. Biomed. Pharmacother., 106, 1586.
32. Altintas, Z., Tothill, I. (2013). Biomarkers and biosensors for the early diagnosis of lung cancer. Sensors Actuators B Chem., 188, 988.
33. Mahato, K., Kumar, A., Maurya, P.K., Chandra, P. (2018). Shifting paradigm of cancer diagnoses in clinically relevant samples based on miniaturized electrochemical nanobiosensors and microfluidic devices. Biosensors and Bioelectronics, 100, 411.
34. Levenson, V.V. (2007). Biomarkers for early detection of breast cancer: What, when, and where? Biochim. Biophys. Acta – Gen. Subj., 1770, 847.
35. Dranoff, G. (2004). Cytokines in cancer pathogenesis and cancer therapy. Nat. Rev. Cancer, 4, 11.
36. Eichbaum, C., Meyer, A.S., Wang, N., Bischofs, E., Steinborn, A., Bruckner, T., Brodt, P., Sohn, C., Eichbaum, M.H.R. (2011). Breast cancer cell-derived cytokines, macrophages and cell adhesion: Implications for metastasis. Anticancer Res., 31, 3219.
37. Song, Q., Merajver, S.D., Li, J.Z. (2015). Cancer classification in the genomic era: Five.
38. Ullah, M.F., Aatif, M. (2009). The footprints of cancer development: cancer biomarkers. Cancer Treat Rev., 35, 193–200.
39. Plummer, M., de Martel, C., Vignat, J., Ferlay, J., Bray, F., Franceschi, S. (2016). Global burden of cancers attributable to infections in 2012: A synthetic analysis. Lancet Glob. Heal., 4, e609–e616.
40. Sholl, L.M., Aisner, D.L., Varella-Garcia, M., Berry, L.D., Dias-Santagata, D., Wistuba, I.I., Chen, H., Fujimoto, J., Kugler, K., Franklin, W.A., et al. (2010).

Biocompatible grapheme oxide-based glucose biosensors. Langmuir, 26, 6158–6160.
41. Massague, J., Obenauf, A.C. (2016). Metastatic colonization by circulating tumour cells. Nature, 529, 298–306.
42. Chang, J.Y., Senan, S., Paul, M.A., Mehran, R.J., Louie, A.V., Balter, P., Groen, H.J.M., McRae, S.E., Widder, J., Feng, L., et al. (2015). Stereotactic ablative radiotherapy versus lobectomy for operable stage I non-small-cell lung cancer: A pooled analysis of two randomised trials. The Lancet Oncology, 16, 630–637.
43. Sohn, T.A., Lillemoe, K.D. (2000). Surgical palliation of pancreatic cancer. Adv. Surg., 34, 249–271.
44. Pannala, R., Basu, A., Petersen, G.M., Chari, S.T. (2009). New-onset diabetes: A potential clue to the early diagnosis of pancreatic cancer. The Lancet Oncology, 10, 88–95.
45. Morganti, A.G., Valentini, V., Macchia, G., Alfieri, S., Trodella, L., Brizi, M.G., et al. (2002). Adjuvant radiotherapy in resectable pancreatic carcinoma. European Journal of Surgical Oncology, 28, 523–530.
46. Molina, R., Barak, V., van Dalen, A., Duffy, M.J., Einarsson, R., Gion, M., et al. (2005). Tumor markers in breast cancer: European Group of Tumor Markers (EGTM) recommendations. Tumor Biology, 26, 281e93.
47. Sturgeon, C.M., Duffy, M.J., Hofmann, B.R., Lamerz, R., Fritsche, H.A., Gaarenstroom, K., et al. (2010). National academy of clinical biochemistry laboratory medicine practice guidelines for use of tumor markers in liver, bladder, cervical, and gastric cancers. Clinical Chemistry, 56, e1e48.
48. Matz, M., Coleman, M.P., Sant, M., Chirlaque, M.D., Visser, O., Gore, M., Allemani, C., Bouzbid, S., Hamdi-Chérif, M., Zaidi, Z. (2017). The histology of ovarian cancer: Worldwide distribution and implications for international survival comparisons (CONCORD-2). Gynecologic Oncol., 144, 405–413.
49. Bast, R.C., Feeney, M., Lazarus, H., Nadler, L., Colvin, R., Knapp, R. (1981). Reactivity of a monoclonal antibody with human ovarian carcinoma. Journal of Clinical Investigation, 68, 1331–1337.
50. Sharma, S.K., Wuest, M., Wang, M., Glubrecht, D., Andrais, B., Lapi, S.E., Wuest, F. (2014). ImmunoPET of epithelial ovarian cancer: Harnessing the potential of CA125 for non-invasive imaging. EJNMMI Research, 4, 60.
51. Hasanzadeh, M., Shadjou, N. (2016). Electrochemical and photoelectrochemical nanoimmunesensing using origami paper based method. Materials Science and Engineering, 61, 979–1001.
52. Hasanzadeh, M., Shadjou, N. (2017). (Nano)-materials and methods of signal enhancement for genosensing of p53 tumor suppressor protein: Novel research overview. Materials Science and Engineering C, 76, 1424–1439.
53. Hasanzadeh, M., Shadjou, N. (2017). What are the reasons for low use of graphene quantum dots in immunosensing of cancer biomarkers? Materials Science and Engineering, 71, 1313–1326.
54. Hasanzadeh, M., Shadjou, N., de la Guardia, M. (2017). Non-invasive diagnosis of oral cancer: The role of electro-analytical methods and nanomaterials. TrAC Trends in Analytical Chemistry, 91, 125–137.
55. Hasanzadeh, M., Shadjou, N., de la Guardia, M. (2017) Current advancement in electrochemical analysis of neurotransmitters in biological fluids. TrAC Trends in Analytical Chemistry, 86, 107–121.

56. Hasanzadeh, M., Shadjou, N., de la Guardia. M. (2017). Aptamer-based assay of biomolecules: Recent advances in electro-analytical approach. Trends in Analytical Chemistry, 89, 119–132.
57. Hasanzadeh, M., Shadjou, N., de la Guardia, M. (2017). Early stage diagnosis of programmed cell death (apoptosis) using electroanalysis: Nanomaterial and methods overview. Trends in Analytical Chemistry, 93, 199–211.
58. Hasanzadeh, M., Shadjou, N., de la Guardia, M. (2018). Cytosensing of cancer cells using antibody-based molecular imprinting: A short-review. TrAC Trends in Analytical Chemistry, 99, 129–134.
59. Hasanzadeh, M., Shadjou, N., de la Guardia, M. (2018). Nanosized hydrophobic gels: Advanced supramolecules for use in electrochemical bio-and immunosensing. TrAC Trends in Analytical Chemistry, 102, 210–224.
60. Razmi, N., Baradaran, B., Hejazi, M., Hasanzadeh, M., Mosafer, J., Mokhtarzadeh, A., de la Guardia, M. (2018). Recent advances on aptamer-based biosensors to detection of platelet-derived growth factor. Biosensors and Bioelectronics, 113, 58–71.
61. Karimzadeh, A., Hasanzadeh, M., Shadjou, N., de la Guardia, M. (2018). Peptide based biosensors. TrAC Trends in Analytical Chemistry, 107, 1–20.
62. Karimzadeh, A., Hasanzadeh, M., Shadjou, N., de la Guardia, M. (2018). Electrochemical biosensing using N-GQDs: Recent advances in analytical approach. TrAC Trends in Analytical Chemistry, 105, 484–491.
63. Siegel, R., Naishadham, D., Jemal, A. (2013). Cancer statistics. CA: A Cancer Journal for Clinicians, 63, 11–30.
64. Labianca, R., Nordlinger, B., Beretta, G.D., Brouquet, A., Cervantes, A. (2010). Primary colon cancer: ESMO clinical practice guidelines for diagnosis, adjuvant treatment and follow-up. Annals of Oncology, 21 (Suppl 5), v70–v77.
65. Berrino, F., De Angelis, R., Sant, M., Rosso, S., Bielska-Lasota, M., Coebergh, J.W., Santaquilani, M. (2007). Survival for eight major cancers and all cancers combined for European adults diagnosed in 1995–99: Results of the EUROCARE-4 study. The Lancet Oncology, 8, 773–783.
66. Lech, G., Slotwinski, R., Krasnodebski, I.W. (2014). The role of tumor markers and biomarkers in colorectal cancer. Neoplasma, 61, 1–8.
67. Lopez-Giacoman, S., Madero, M. (2015). Biomarkers in chronic kidney disease, from kidney function to kidney damage. World Journal of Nephrology, 4, 57–73.
68. Tan, H., Xu, J., Liu, Y. (2022). Ageing, cellular senescence and chronic kidney disease: Experimental evidence. Current Opinion in Nephrology and Hypertension, 31, 235–243.
69. Couser, W.G., Remuzzi, G., Mendis, S., Tonelli, M.J.K.I. (2011). The contribution of chronic kidney disease to the global burden of major noncommunicable diseases. Kidney International, 80, 1258–1270.
70. Hassan, A., Khalaily, N., Kilav-Levin, R., Nechama, M., Volovelsky, O., Silver, J., Naveh-Many, T. (2022). Molecular mechanisms of parathyroid disorders in chronic kidney disease. Metabolites, 12, 1.
71. Pradeepa, R., Mohan, V. (2021). Epidemiology of type 2 diabetes in India. Indian Journal of Ophthalmology, 69, 2932–2938.
72. Mizdrak, M., Kumric, M., Kurir, T.T., Bozic, J. (2022). Emerging biomarkers for early detection of chronic kidney disease. Journal of Personalized Medicine, 12, 548.

73. Hernandez-Ramirez, D., Mendoza-Huizar, L.H., Galan-Vidal, C.A., Aguilar-Lira, G.Y., Alvarez-Romero, G.A. (2022). Review-trends in the development of non-enzymatic electrochemical sensors modified with a metal-organic framework for quantification of uric acid. Journal of the Electrochemical Society, 169, 057522.
74. Roopa, R.A., Mantelingu, K., Guin, M., Thimmaiah, S.B. (2022). Bienzymatic spectrophotometric method for uric acid estimation in human serum and urine. Journal of Analytical Chemistry, 77, 301–307.
75. Liu, J., Xu, C., Ying, L., Zang, S., Zhuang, Z., Lv, H., Yang, W., Luo, Y., Ma, X., Wang, L., et al. (2017). Relationship of serum uric acid level with non-alcoholic fatty liver disease and its inflammation progression in non-obese adults. Hepatology Research, 47, E104–E112.
76. Mitsudomi, T., Kosaka, T., Endoh, H., Horio, Y., Hida, T., Mori, S., Hatooka, S., Shinoda, M., Takahashi, T., Yatabe, Y. (2005). Mutations of the epidermal growth factor receptor gene predict prolonged survival after gefitinib treatment in patients with non-small-cell lung cancer with postoperative recurrence. Journal of Clinical Oncology, 23, 2513–2520.
77. Nicolini, A., Ferrari, P., Duffy, M.J. (2018). Prognostic and predictive biomarkers in breast cancer: Past, present and future. Seminars in Cancer Biology, 52, 56.
78. Armstrong, A.J., Eisenberger, M.A., Halabi, S., Oudard, S., Nanus, D.M., Petrylak, D.P., Sartor, A.O., Scher, H.I. (2012). Biomarkers in the Management and Treatment of Men with Metastatic Castration-Resistant Prostate Cancer. European Urology, 61, 549–559.

4

MXene-Based Emerging 2D Materials for Biomedical Photothermal and Photodynamic Therapeutic Applications

Kajal Yadav, Kamna Chaturvedi, Anju Singhwane, and Sarika Verma

4.1 Introduction

Nanomedicine advancements have spurred exploration into diverse treatment methods, with phototherapy gaining notable attention due to its minimal invasiveness, exceptional tumor selectivity, precise spatial and temporal control, and minimal toxicity. Photodynamic therapy and photothermal therapy stand out as the primary categories of phototherapy [1]. A wide array of innovative inorganic nanosystems has emerged in the evolving landscape of biomedicine and nanobiotechnology. These nanosystems offer the possibility of multiple theranostic approaches, including synergistic therapy and multimodal imaging, presenting promising alternatives for addressing various diseases [2]. Recent studies have extensively explored the function of nanoparticles (NPs) in diagnosing and curing various diseases including antimicrobial systems. One of the key objectives of employing nanotechnology in bacterial infection treatment is the development of precise NPs that can effectively target specific cells. NPs offer several advantages, including their gradual degradation, controlled-release capabilities, superior surface performance, and high optical absorption. These attributes make NPs valuable agents for techniques such as photothermal therapy (PTT) and photodynamic therapy (PDT). Consequently, integrating NPs into these therapeutic approaches enhances treatment efficiency while concurrently reducing potential side effects [3]. Light-based treatments, such as photothermal and photodynamic therapy, have been harnessed as minimally invasive methods for targeting and eliminating various bacterial infections. These modalities can eradicate infection while causing minimal harm to surrounding healthy tissues. Furthermore, advancing methods mediated by light involving

DOI: 10.1201/9781003353287-4

photosensitizers and nanoparticles as therapeutic and diagnostic agents hold significant promise in pursuing effective treatment [4].

The uncontrolled proliferation of harmful bacteria represents a significant global challenge, posing a substantial threat to public health. This issue ultimately leads to economic burdens on infected individuals and society [5]. Infectious bacteria consistently result in wound infections [6] and transmission of diseases [7]. Undoubtedly, the rise of bacterial resistance to drugs and the development of biofilms contribute to severe biological crises. Therefore, the pursuit of innovative, effective treatment methods that do not trigger drug resistance holds immense importance in addressing these challenges. Non-invasive photothermal therapy activated by light irradiation and photodynamic therapy shows great potential as substitutes for antibiotics in combating bacterial growth [8]. Utilizing hyperthermia levels surpassing bacterial tolerance, this therapy can effectively and controllably compromise the integrity of pathogenic bacteria [9]. Numerous antibiotic-free approaches have been adopted for addressing bacterial infections, employing diverse methodologies, including releasing metallic ions [10]. Within these approaches, near-infrared light-based phototherapy, encompassing both photodynamic and photothermal therapy, stands out as an exceptionally promising therapeutic strategy. Its attributes include profound tissue penetration, assured biosafety, and swift, highly efficient therapeutic efficacy devoid of bacterial resistance [11].

Many materials exhibiting photothermal properties have been harnessed and engineered, encompassing materials derived from carbon [12], noble metal nanoparticles [13], and metal–organic frameworks [14]. MXenes have emerged as standout candidates within these options owing to their remarkable characteristics: an atomic-thin structure with a high aspect ratio, superb photothermal capabilities, minimal toxicity, and outstanding ability to disperse in water [15]. MXenes are a diverse category of two-dimensional (2D) materials composed of carbides, carbonitrides, and nitrides of transition metals generally denoted by the chemical formula Mn+1XnTx [16]. The 2D materials within this group showcase strong light-absorption capabilities throughout the spectrum, spanning ultraviolet, visible, and near-infrared spectra. This quality demonstrates their substantial promise in photoenergy conversion applications [17]. MXenes possess inherent photothermal and photodynamic capabilities, enabling them to function directly as photothermal agents or photosensitizers by utilizing their photo-responsive building units [18]. MXenes, characterized by minimal cytotoxicity and excellent biocompatibility, serve as exceptional systems for in vivo therapeutic applications. They demonstrate potential in various applications, including treating bacterial infections and facilitating the formation of granulation tissue. This significantly enhances the therapeutic effectiveness compared to traditional bandages [19].

In the last decade, there have been substantial efforts devoted to formulating antimicrobial materials based on MXenes. These materials are designed to exhibit photothermal therapy. In this chapter, we initially provide a comprehensive overview and introduction to the synthetic procedures and textural characteristics of MXenes. Subsequently, we provide a comprehensive summary and analysis of the antibacterial mechanisms, primarily focusing on their intrinsic photothermal therapy and other synergistic PDT. MXenes have surfaced as a promising agent in antibacterial therapy through their application in photodynamic and photothermal therapy [20–26]. MXenes exhibit strong light-to-heat conversion properties, raising temperatures in targeted areas, thereby effectively destroying bacterial cells. Their dual functionality in PDT and PTT makes MXenes versatile and potent agents in combating bacterial infections.

4.2 Synthesis Methods of MXenes

MXenes, a class of two-dimensional materials, are primarily synthesized through targeted removal of the 'A' layers from MAX phases. Various synthesis approaches have been developed to produce MXenes with tailored properties, involving key steps of exfoliating MAX phases and subsequent layer separation. Commonly employed methods include the following.

4.2.1 Chemical Etching

This involves the use of strong etchants (e.g., hydrofluoric acid, hydrogen chloride) to selectively remove the 'A' layers from MAX phases, leading to the formation of multilayered MXene precursors [27].

4.2.2 Intercalation and Delamination

The precursor MXene layers are intercalated with specific agents to facilitate delamination and exfoliation as shown in Figure 4.1, producing few-layer or single-layer MXenes [28].

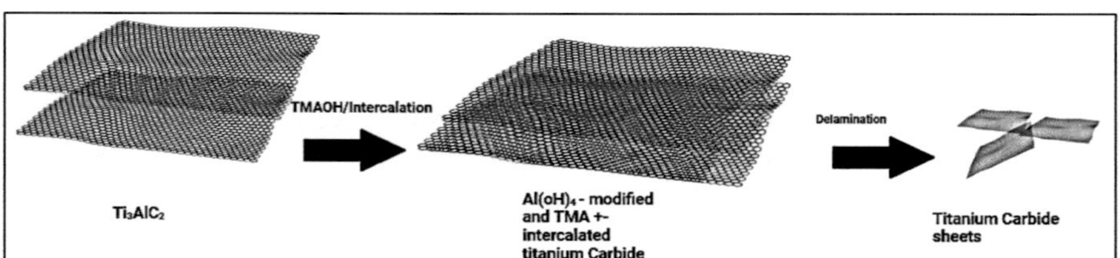

FIGURE 4.1
Illustrative diagram depicting the intercalation and delamination processes of MXene [29].

4.2.3 In situ Synthesis

This study introduced an innovative single-step in situ method involving a reaction with molten $SnCl_2$ salt and Ti_3AlC_2 to synthesize composites of $Ti_3C_2T_x$ MXene confined within Sn nanoparticles. Throughout the synthetic procedure, $SnCl_2$ served as more than just a Lewis acid, playing a role in etching Ti_3AlC_2 and generating MXene but also underwent an in situ transformation into Sn nanoparticles that became confined within the layers of MXene [30].

4.2.4 Surface Functionalization

This study delved into exploring the capacity to adjust the MXene's work function $Ti_3C_2T_x$—where T_x signifies surface termination—synthesized via two methods: the traditional hydrogen fluoride etched route and the newly devised molten salt-etched method. Upon subjecting MXene samples to gas-phase reactions, significant work function (WF) variations surpassing 0.6 eV are attained, demonstrating the possibility of exact control over the WF. Notably, the WF experienced an increase from approximately ~4.23 eV (in N-doped MXene synthesized using molten salt etching) to ~4.85 eV (in N-doped MXene synthesized using HF etching) [31].

4.3 Use of MXenes in Photothermal and Photodynamic Therapeutic Applications

The adaptable 2D nanostructure within MXenes, coupled with their modifiable chemical compositions, grants them diverse properties that prove advantageous in biomedical applications. Thus far, researchers have harnessed these multifunctional 2D MXenes and their combinations for theranostic purposes, encompassing phototherapy such as photothermal therapy (PTT), combined photothermal/photodynamic/chemotherapies, and antimicrobial applications. In this section, we present an overview of the manifold uses of different types of 2D MXene materials in PDT and PTT [32].

4.3.1 Photothermal Therapy

Biophotonic nanomedicines are made possible by the unique potential of light-interacting nanomaterials [33]. Multifunctional nanoparticles could be the basis for developing image-guided therapies [34]. Photothermal antibacterial therapy synergistically eliminates bacteria by leveraging high temperatures. This approach capitalizes on the collective benefits: PTT induces local hyperthermia, reducing cellular activity. Ultimately, this mechanism works in

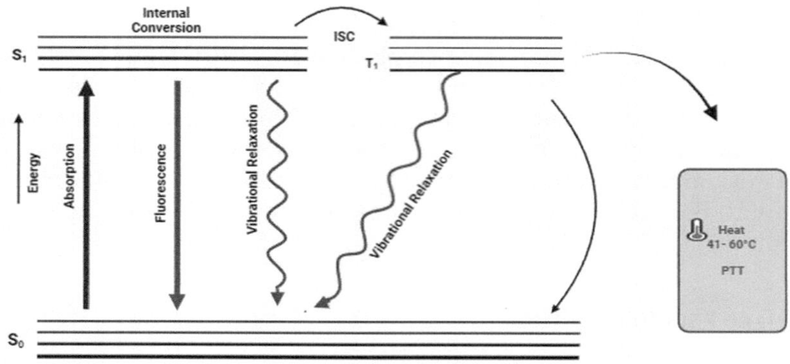

FIGURE 4.2
Systematic illustration of photothermal therapy including electron transfer after getting near-infrared light.

tandem to effectively deactivate and eliminate bacterial cells [35]. PTT uses the heat generated when nanocomposites are exposed to near-infrared radiation (NIR) to destroy bacterial cells [33]. Photothermal processes describe the inclination of a light-absorbing substance to release electronic excitation energy by swiftly transferring it through vibrational modes, thereby causing a rise in the kinetic energy of the surrounding molecules or particles near the light-absorbing center essentially, as predicted in Figure 4.2, generating localized heat [36]. Elevated temperatures, resulting in increased thermal energy, can cause harm to various structural elements within cells, such as proteins and DNA damage. This cumulative damage ultimately results in the demise of cells [37]. Cell death through the photothermal effect is induced using the near-infrared region, which spans from 800 to 2500 nm [38]. PTT employs elevated levels of light energy to attain temperatures within the range of 43–55°C for sub-coagulative effects or 55–100°C for coagulative effects [39]. In recent studies, emerging PTT has garnered significant interest due to its remarkable effectiveness in treating cancer. This approach involves deploying a nanomaterial with photothermal properties, known as a photothermal agent (PAT), to the site. Importantly, this technique allows for precise targeting of the area while preserving the health of surrounding tissues, minimizing collateral damage [40].

Two fundamental parameters primarily influence photothermal agents' performance in PTT. The first parameter is their capacity for absorbing light, quantified by the extinction coefficient (ε). The second parameter relates to their effectiveness in producing heat upon exposure to external light, referred to as photothermal conversion efficiency (PCE or η) [41]. Numerous nanomaterials have demonstrated potential for PTT, offering promising options for various biomedical applications. Some notable nanomaterials in PTT include gold nanorods, copper sulfide nanoparticles, black phosphorus, and MXenes. MXenes, in particular, have shown significant potential for deep-tissue PTT due to their exceptional photothermal properties and NIR absorption. Researchers continue to explore and develop these nanomaterials for in vivo PTT applications to improve cancer therapy and other medical treatments [40]. MXenes possess several advantages, such as their inherent two-dimensional structure, effective confinement and conversion of electromagnetic waves, and the ability to harness the localized surface plasmon resonance (LSPR) effect. These characteristics collectively bestow upon MXenes a remarkable capacity for photoenergy conversion, leading to exceptional photo-induced antimicrobial effects [42].

4.3.2 Photothermal Antimicrobial Mechanism

Exposing bacteria to temperatures exceeding 45°C leads to a significant change in their viability; various photothermal agents can induce distinct mechanisms of photothermal conversion. These mechanisms include localized surface plasmon resonance in metals, the generation and relaxation of electron–hole pairs in semiconductors, as well as the excitation of HOMO (highest occupied molecular orbital)–LUMO (lowest unoccupied molecular orbital) and the vibration of molecular lattices, depending on the specific PTAs utilized [43]. The photothermal antibacterial action of nanoparticles (NPs) relies on their ability to absorb visible light radiation, forming plasmons—collective oscillations of conduction electrons. Subsequently, the generated heat is rapidly transferred to the bacteria in the vicinity, causing cell or bacteria death. Several factors, including the size, shape, and dielectric constant of the NPs, the permittivity of the surrounding materials, the wavelength of the incident light, and the intensity of light, influence the effectiveness of photothermal bacterial ablation. Adjusting these parameters allows for the optimization of photothermal interactions. Materials produce a photothermal effect by instigating the vibration of their molecular lattice. When exposed to light energy, an electron within the material transitioning from its ground state (LUMO) to a higher-energy orbital (HOMO) progresses. Subsequently, the relaxation of these higher excitation states back to lower-energy states is facilitated by electron–phonon coupling.

Consequently, the deriving energy from the electrons after excitement is transferred to vibrational patterns within the lattice of atoms, resulting in an elevation of temperature [44]. The photothermal effect cannot be considered independently of other mechanisms involved in antimicrobial action. These include nano-perforation, destabilization of membranes, binding with biomolecules, and causing oxidative damage [45]. The interactions between NPs and bacteria are contingent upon several factors, including the surface chemistry, charge, and hydrophobicity of the NPs. Primarily, the effectiveness of photothermal action relies on the dielectric constants of the photothermal agent nanoparticles and the materials in their proximity [46].

4.3.3 Photothermal Conversion Mechanism of MXene

The photothermal effect is described by a rise in temperature in a material resulting from light absorption. Nanostructured photothermal materials uniquely confine this effect to extremely small regions, down to the nanoscale. This phenomenon is governed by the diverse ways different materials interact with light, closely tied to their intrinsic electronic properties or bandgap structures. These variations in light–matter interactions give rise to distinct photothermal conversion mechanisms [47]. Research on photothermally active MXenes is still underway, so the underlying mechanism remains incompletely understood. Numerous ground-breaking studies have been conducted to elucidate this mechanism [43]. Some studies have revealed that MXenes exhibit an electromagnetic interference (EMI) effect. In this phenomenon, electromagnetic waves not reflected at the MXene lattice structure can penetrate and experience internal reflections within the layers. Ultimately, these waves are absorbed within the MXene structure with minimal emission. This unique property ensures potential light absorption across a wide solar spectrum range for MXene compounds [48]. According to some researchers, the photothermal conversion mechanism of Ti_3C_2 is attributed to the LSPR effect [49]. Researchers have showcased the potential of plasmonic systems to generate LSPR-induced hot electrons. These hot electrons can be harnessed for the conversion of energy and storage when coupled with electron-accepting semiconductor materials [50]. Exfoliated MXene nanosheets with exceptionally high metallic conductivity are 'semimetal' and have a property similar to that of metals. They are derived from MAX ceramics. MXenes are unique; they combine characteristics of both ceramics and metals, thanks to incorporating carbon atoms within the metal lattice. It has been noted that only Ti_3C_2 flake films can achieve remarkably high electrical conductivity, reaching values of approximately $\approx 4600 \pm 1100$ S cm^{-1} [51]. Research has shown that absorbing bands of the PEG/Ti_3C_2 composite in the visible and near-infrared spectral regions were intensified as a product of the LSPR effect induced by Ti_3C_2. This enhancement in absorption is advantageous for efficient solar energy capture and rapid conversion for photothermal applications and storage [49]. The absorption spectra of ultrathin Ti_3C_2 nanosheets were measured in research described by Lin. Ti_3C_2 nanosheets exhibited robust absorption within the near-infrared (NIR) region, specifically in the range of 750–850 nm, which is reminiscent of absorption behavior seen in specific noble metal nanoparticles that exhibit the LSPR effect, such as Au NPs [52]. It has been confirmed that arrays of nano-sized disks composed of MXene demonstrate robust LSPR at NIR frequencies, leading to a broad absorption spectrum. This unique combination of strong absorption light and the LSPR effect shows MXene materials to have outstanding photothermal conversion capabilities. This includes the efficient capture of solar energy and the subsequent storage and utilization of the converted thermal energy [53].

4.3.4 Photothermal Conversion Efficiency of MXene

Carbon-based materials have been extensively explored and designed for their photothermal properties because of their versatility and distinct properties. MXenes have become exceptional photothermal materials due to their remarkable characteristics, including atomic-thin thickness, high aspect ratio, outstanding photothermal efficiency, lower toxicity, and exceptional dispersibility in aqueous solutions [54]. MXenes constitute a diverse group of two-dimensional materials consisting of nitrides, transition metal carbides, carbonitrides, and nitrides, generally identified by the chemical formula Mn+1XnTx [16]. These 2D materials exhibit robust light-absorption capabilities that span the entire spectrum, near-infrared, ultraviolet (UV), and near-infrared (NIR) spectra. As a result, they hold significant promise for various applications in photonic energy conversion [55].

Researchers have achieved significant breakthroughs in advancing MXene materials for PTT in the past few years. Notably, Nb2C has originated as a promising candidate with exceptionally elevated photothermal conversion efficiency, exhibiting effectiveness in both the NIR-I and NIR-II regions [56]. Ta4C3Tx-SP nanosheets have been developed to use dual-mode imaging simultaneously using PA and CT to visualize tumors within living organisms [57]. Moreover, advancements have been made in developing MQDs (metal-quantum dots) with exceptionally high photothermal conversion efficiency [58].

Furthermore, Shao et al. explored the synthesis of nitride-based MXenes and quantum dots. Such quantum dots showed exceptional high photothermal conversion efficiency observed in both the first and second near-infrared biological windows (NIR-I, 48.62% at 808 nm; NIR-II, 45.51% at 1064 nm), Furthermore to their favorable biocompatibility and efficient photothermal therapeutic capabilities, Ti2NTx quantum dots also demonstrated appropriate degradability and rate of excretion in vivo. After exerting their photothermal therapeutic effects, these quantum dots could be smoothly eliminated from the body [59].

4.3.5 Photothermal Antibacterial Therapy by MXene-Based Materials

Two-dimensional MXenes, a recent class of materials, have showcased impressive PCE compared to the materials mentioned earlier. This heightened PCE is attributable to their remarkable absorption of light capabilities in the NIR range, suggesting that MXenes can serve as highly efficient photothermal agents [56]. As an example, $Ti_3C_2T_x$, recognized as one of the initial and most extensively employed MXenes, has demonstrated notable attributes such as high effectiveness, requiring minimal dosage, and rapid action in its

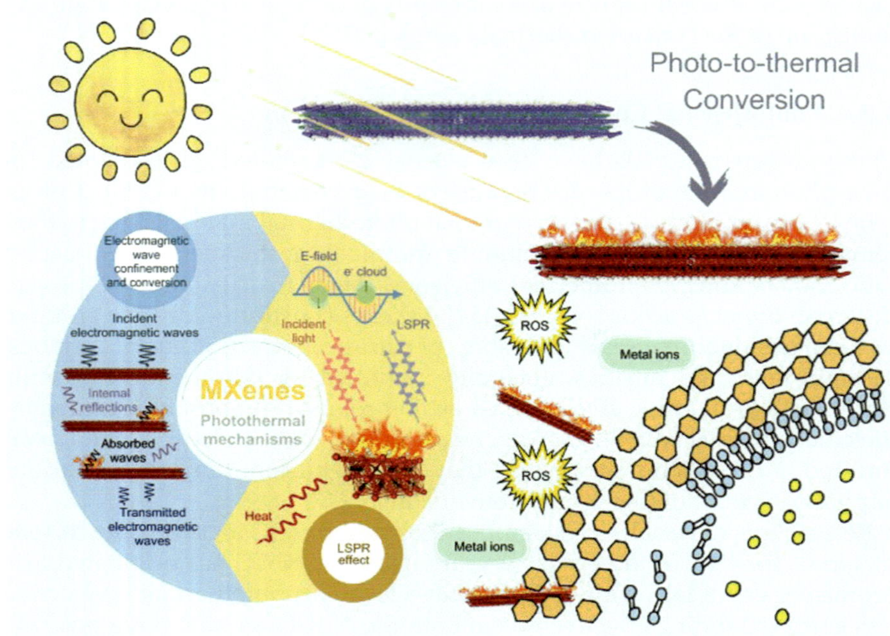

FIGURE 4.3
Demonstration of MXene-based photothermal therapy leading to cell death [29].

antibacterial applications [60]. Under the influence of photothermal therapy, $Ti_3C_2T_x$ disrupted the protective membrane and swiftly deactivated the inherent bioactive matrix, as shown in Figure 4.3 When subjected to 808-nm near-infrared light irradiation, notable antibacterial effects became evident in a solution containing $Ti_3C_2T_x$ nanosheets within just 20 minutes [61]. A notable case study highlighted the utilization of $Ag/Ti_3C_2T_x$ for a synergistic antibacterial effect. This study initially adsorbed silver ions onto negatively charged $Ti_3C_2T_x$ nanosheets which were reduced by sodium citrate, producing $Ag/Ti_3C_2T_x$ composites. A suspension of $Ag/Ti_3C_2T_x$ at a concentration of 200 micrograms per milliliter exhibited limited antibacterial activity without light. However, these composites effectively eradicated all bacteria upon exposure to 808-nm NIR light irradiation. The scanning electron microscopy results aligned with the antibacterial tests, illustrating noticeable synergistic antibacterial performance exhibited by $Ag/Ti_3C_2T_x$ under NIR irradiation. High-resolution imaging revealed cytoplasm leakage and cytolysis in bacteria exposed to light. The primary factor influencing the antimicrobial efficacy of silver nanoparticles could be the release of Ag^+ ions [62]. In this study, they immersed a thin film comprising $Ag/Ti_3C_2T_x$ in a specific quantity of solution and exposed it to irradiation from Xe lamp (500 W, 31.45 W cm^{-2}) under light exposure, and the concentration of silver ions that were released was measured at 0.46 mg mL^{-1}, nearly 300 times higher compared to the control group. This observation suggested that the release of Ag ions was triggered by light, consequently amplifying the antimicrobial efficacy of the composite [63]. In a recent investigation, Li fabricated NIR-responsive MXenes/CuS composites via a reaction between C_2H_5NS and Cu^{2+} ions adsorbed onto the outer layer of $Ti_3C_2T_x$. This method enabled the regulated discharge of Cu^{2+} , SEM images revealed uniform growth of CuS nanoparticles, ranging in diameter from 100 to 500 nm, on the surface of multilayered $Ti_3C_2T_x$. Under NIR light exposure, the liberation of Cu^{2+} ions was notably enhanced. Due to combined contributions arising from the photothermal effects of MXenes and CuS, including contributions of the PT effects of CuS and MXenes, the antibacterial efficacy of the MXenes/CuS composite surpassed 99% against both *E. coli* and *S. aureus* [64].

4.3.6 Photodynamic Therapy

Photodynamic therapy utilizes light-responsive substances to produce reactive oxygen species (ROS). This, in turn, has the potential to oxidize neighboring biomolecules, such as nucleic acids, proteins, and lipids, resulting in substantial harm to the targeted cells [65]. First, the process starts with administering a photosensitizer, a light-sensitive drug, and exposing it to light with a specific wavelength matching the photosensitizer's absorption range. This process triggers the generation of cytotoxic free radicals due to oxygen in the tissue, leading to the immediate eradication of tumor cells, destruction of the microvascular structure, and activation of inflammatory reactions at designated treatment sites [66]. These photosensitizers (PSs) remain inert in the absence of light and pose no toxicity concerns until light induced by the laser activates them. This triggering takes place in the presence of oxygen, commonly under visible light, frequently making use of long-wavelength red light. Following this phenomenon, the photosensitizer conveys energy to molecular oxygen, resulting in damage to targeted cells. The photochemical interaction with oxygen induces the production of reactive oxygen species (ROS). The interaction between ROS and oxygen results in the production of the superoxide anion (O_{2-}). Cytotoxic singlet oxygen is produced from the interaction of PS with triplet oxygen ($3O_2$). The superoxide anion and singlet oxygen contribute to cell death through two mechanisms: the first involves direct pathways such as necrosis and apoptosis. In contrast, the second mechanism encompasses indirect pathways, entailing microvascular complications [67].

A specific wavelength of light is directed at the tumorous region where the photosensitizer has ideally accumulated, allowing for the initiation of type 1 and type 2 reactions induced by light. In PDT, these reactions generate ROS, ultimately causing tissue destruction [68]. Photodynamic therapy can

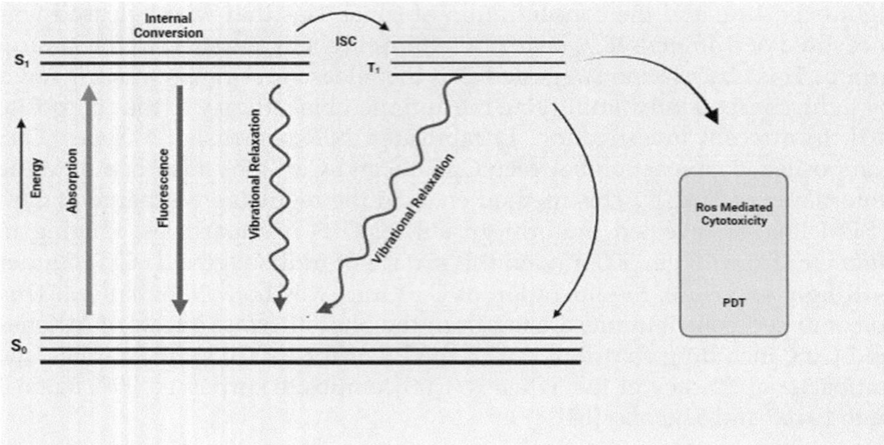

FIGURE 4.4
Systematic representation of photodynamic therapy including Jablonski diagram.

be designated into two types, namely, type 1 PDT and type 2 PDT, based on mechanisms of ROS generation [69]. In the context of type 1 PDT, when the PS is exposed to irradiation, the energy absorbed by ground-state PS transitions to a singlet state. These singlet PS molecules, either by producing fluorescence or non-radiative decay, return to their ground state. Alternatively, they can undergo intersystem crossing (ISC), transitioning to a longer-lived triplet state. In this triplet state, the photosensitizer can transfer protons or electrons to substrates, like cell membranes or molecules rich in electrons, as depicted in Figure 4.4 [70]. Radicals generated in this process are both short-lived and exceptionally reactive. They engage with oxygen and water molecules, resulting in the production of superoxide anion, hydroxyl radicals, and hydrogen peroxide [69]. This causes particular damage to biomolecules and starts a series of radical reactions [71]. Triplet PS energy is transferred to triplet oxygen ($3O_2$) in type II PDT, producing cytotoxic singlet oxygen. This singlet oxygen selectively interacts with cellular components, including the nucleus, cell membrane, endoplasmic reticulum, lysosomes, and nucleus, ultimately leading to cell death. The photosensitizer's type and concentration will determine whether type 1 and type 2 processes can occur [70]. Type I reactions frequently result in more extensive damage. In type I PDT, photosensitizers are consumed, requiring regeneration [71].

Traditional type II PDT holds significant promise for anticancer treatment, but its efficiency is significantly impeded by hypoxia. Innovative PDT approaches have emerged to address this challenge, including fractional photodynamic therapy, type I photodynamic therapy, remote-controlled release of singlet oxygen ($1O_2$), and multimodal therapy [72].

4.3.7 Photodynamic Antibacterial Therapy by MXene-Based Materials

The restricted bandgap of the $Ti_3C_2T_x$ nanosheets (approximately 1.69 eV) significantly impedes their efficiency by causing swift recombination of electron–hole pairs generated through photon absorption, consequently restricting the release of reactive oxygen species [73]. Zhu B et al.'s study involved the creation of Ti_3C_2@gold nanorods (GNRs)/PDA nanoparticles demonstrating combined photodynamic antibacterial characteristics. This was accomplished through the application of a polydopamine (PDA) coating on the surface of in situ grown Ti_3C_2@GNRs. The aggregation of Ti_3C_2 MXene nanosheets was effectively hindered by the growth of gold nanorods, thereby ensuring the unique photodynamic antibacterial efficacy exhibited by Ti_3C_2. Furthermore, these nanoparticles exhibited synergistically enhanced photodynamic properties attributed to the notable photodynamic characteristics of Ti_3C_2 MXene and PDA. Consequently, the minimum inhibitory concentrations of Ti_3C_2@GNRs/PDA50 nanoparticles against *E. coli* and *S. aureus* were diminished to around 0.07 mg/mL. This study utilizes the $^1O_2$-generating potential of Ti_3C_2 MXene and PDA to create Ti_3C_2@GNRs/PDA nanoparticles, demonstrating synergistically enhanced photodynamic antibacterial effects. Such advancements hold promise for applications in antibiotic-free antibacterial fields [74].

Feng H et al. created environmentally friendly antibacterial materials with broad-spectrum and long-lasting effectiveness. Ternary composites of BiOI@Bi_2S_3/MXene showcase both PTT and PDT for antibacterial applications. These composites' synthesis involved in situ vulcanization to create hollow flower-shaped BiOI on the surface of two-dimensional Ti_3C_2 MXene. The distinctive structure of hollow flower-shaped BiOI, exposing a significant portion of the (001) crystal plane, intensifies light reflection and scattering. This configuration provides more active sites, enhancing light utilization. Under 808-nm irradiation, these composites exhibited a photothermal conversion efficiency of 57.8% markedly enhancing the PTT antibacterial efficacy. Crucially, the enhanced bacteriostatic performance of PDT was achieved through the promotion of charge transfer and the reduction of electron–hole recombination at the heterogeneous interface [75]. Wang et al. developed photothermal–photodynamic Ti_3C_2 nanosheets, obtained through TMAOH-driven intercalation and delamination, that exhibit higher synergistic antibacterial efficiency than Ti_3C_2 nanosheets obtained through the conventional exfoliation methods involving HF or in situ HF (HCl + LiF). Moreover, the antibacterial mechanism elucidates the disruption of biofilms, and the release of bacterial contents and permeability plays a substantial role in the ROS reaction and photothermal antibacterial activity when exposed to NIR irradiation after Ti_3C_2 nanosheets adhering to the target bacteria, as shown in Figure 4.5 [76].

Numerous studies have demonstrated that when MXene is used as a photosensitizer, it may develop ROS when exposed to particular wavelengths

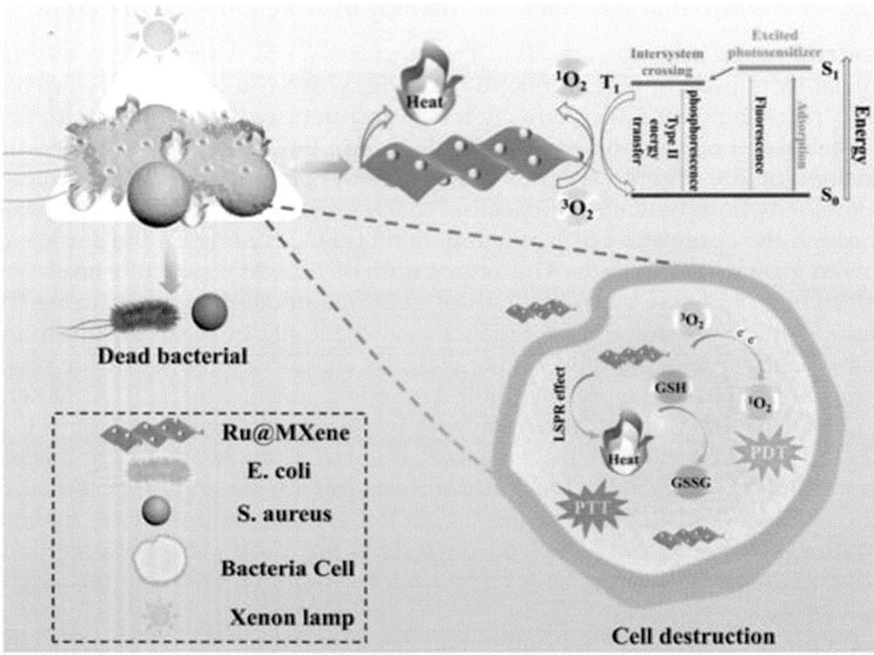

FIGURE 4.5
A schematic illustration depicting the utilization of Ru@MXene as a photoconverting agent designed for the generation of heat and singlet oxygen ($1O_2$), aimed at achieving combined photothermal (PTT) and photodynamic (PDT) antibacterial activities [77].

of light, a crucial aspect of cancer treatment. As research advances, more MXene variants are being recognized for their potential in photodynamic therapy [40].

4.4 Conclusion and Future Perspectives

MXenes have arisen as highly assuring materials in biological applications in recent years. Owing to their diverse chemical compositions, unique morphologies, and impressive electrical conductivities, MXenes present compelling opportunities for various biological applications. Notably, when combined with ceramics, polymers, carbon, and metal-based nanocomposites, they form exceptional composites that exhibit enhanced properties. Using MXene materials in photothermal and photodynamic therapies is a promising development in antibacterial therapy. MXenes provide a unique combination of properties for the efficient and targeted destruction of bacterial cells due to their high photothermal conversion efficiency and capacity to produce ROS. These treatments are safer and more potent because they have demonstrated great promise in selectively eliminating bacterial cells while minimizing harm to healthy tissues. The versatility of MXenes makes them useful tools for upcoming biomedical applications because of their tunable nature, which enables customization to meet particular treatment requirements. MXene-based photothermal and photodynamic antibacterial therapies will likely play an increasingly significant role as research advances, ultimately raising the quality of life of countless patients.

The potential for MXene-based photodynamic and photothermal therapy to revolutionize the treatment of cancer and various other medical conditions is extremely promising. The family of 2D transition metal nitrides and carbides called MXenes has already demonstrated remarkable qualities like high surface area, exceptional biocompatibility, and excellent electrical conductivity. Because of these qualities, they are the perfect candidates for creating cutting-edge PTT and PDT platforms. We can expect significant advancements in MXene-based therapeutics in the upcoming years, with researchers concentrating on MXene nanosheet optimization for effective light absorption and conversion and customizing their surface chemistry to improve targeting and drug-delivery capabilities.

Combining MXene-based PTT and PDT with cutting-edge innovations like precision medicine and immunotherapy may reveal new synergistic strategies for highly effective and individualized cancer treatments. We anticipate a time when MXene-based PTT and PDT will play a critical role in minimally invasive, highly targeted, and precisely controlled cancer treatments, ultimately enhancing patient quality of life and outcomes. This is due to our growing understanding of MXenes and the advancement of their synthesis techniques.

References

1. Naief MF, Mohammed SN, Mayouf HJ, Mohammed AM. A review of the role of carbon nanotubes for cancer treatment based on photothermal and photodynamic therapy techniques. Journal of Organometallic Chemistry. 2023 Jul 20; 999(15 October 2023):122819.
2. Fan T, Yan L, He S, Hong Q, Ai F, He S, Ji T, Hu X, Ha E, Zhang B, Li Z. Biodistribution, degradability and clearance of 2D materials for their biomedical applications. Chemical Society Reviews. 2022; 51: 7732.
3. Sargazi S, Simge ER, Gelen SS, Rahdar A, Bilal M, Arshad R, Ajalli N, Khan MF, Pandey S. Application of titanium dioxide nanoparticles in photothermal and photodynamic therapy of cancer: An updated and comprehensive review.

Journal of Drug Delivery Science and Technology. 2022 Jul 19; 75(September 2022): 103605.
4. Kadkhoda J, Tarighatnia A, Barar J, Aghanejad A, Davaran S. Recent advances and trends in nanoparticles based photothermal and photodynamic therapy. Photodiagnosis and Photodynamic Therapy. 2022 Mar 1;37:102697.
5. Tavakolian M, Jafari SM, van de Ven TG. A review on surface-functionalized cellulosic nanostructures as biocompatible antibacterial materials. Nano-Micro Letters. 2020 Dec;12:1–23.
6. Karner L, Drechsler S, Metzger M, Slezak P, Zipperle J, Pinar G, Sterflinger K, Leisch F, Grillari J, Osuchowski M, Dungel P. Contamination of wounds with fecal bacteria in immuno-suppressed mice. Scientific Reports. 2020 Jul 13;10(1):11494.
7. Gao H, Cui C, Wang L, Jacobs-Lorena M, Wang S. Mosquito microbiota and implications for disease control. Trends in Parasitology. 2020 Feb 1;36(2):98–111.
8. Li J, Li Z, Liu X, Li C, Zheng Y, Yeung KW, Cui Z, Liang Y, Zhu S, Hu W, Qi Y. Interfacial engineering of $Bi_2S_3/Ti_3C_2T_x$ MXene based on work function for rapid photo-excited bacteria-killing. Nature Communications. 2021 Feb 22;12(1):1224.
9. Cai X, Tian J, Zhu J, Chen J, Li L, Yang C, Chen J, Chen D. Photodynamic and photothermal co-driven CO-enhanced multi-mode synergistic antibacterial nanoplatform to effectively fight against biofilm infections. Chemical Engineering Journal. 2021 Dec 15;426:131919.
10. Xiong K, Li J, Tan L, Cui Z, Li Z, Wu S, Liang Y, Zhu S, Liu X. Ag_2S decorated nanocubes with enhanced near-infrared photothermal and photodynamic properties for rapid sterilization. Colloid and Interface Science Communications. 2019 Nov 1;33:100201.
11. H, Wang W, Zhang M, Zhu S, Wang Q, Liu J, Chen S. 2D titanium carbide-based nanocomposites for photocatalytic bacteriostatic applications. Applied Catalysis B: Environmental. 2020 Jun 5;266:118609.
12. Yang Y, Zhou X, Chan YK, Wang Z, Li L, Li J, Liang K, Deng Y. Photo-activated nanofibrous membrane with self-rechargeable antibacterial function for stubborn infected cutaneous regeneration. Small. 2022 Mar;18(12):2105988.
13. Yu Z, Jiang L, Liu R, Zhao W, Yang Z, Zhang J, Jin S. Versatile self-assembled MXene-Au nanocomposites for SERS detection of bacteria, antibacterial and photothermal sterilization. Chemical Engineering Journal. 2021 Dec 15;426:131914.
14. Yang Y, Deng Y, Huang J, Fan X, Cheng C, Nie C, Ma L, Zhao W, Zhao C. Size-transformable metal–organic framework–derived nanocarbons for localized chemo-photothermal bacterial ablation and wound disinfection. Advanced Functional Materials. 2019 Aug;29(33):1900143.
15. Chaturvedi K, Hada V, Paul S, Sarma B, Malvi D, Dhangar M, Bajpai H, Singhwane A, Srivastava AK, Verma S. The rise of MXene: A wonder 2D material, from its synthesis and properties to its versatile applications—A comprehensive review. Topics in Current Chemistry. 2023 Mar;381(2):11.
16. Naguib M, Mochalin VN, Barsoum MW, Gogotsi Y. 25th anniversary article: MXenes: A new family of two-dimensional materials. Advanced Materials. 2014 Feb;26(7):992–1005.

17. Xiang Z, Shi Y, Zhu X, Cai L, Lu W. Flexible and waterproof 2D/1D/0D construction of MXene-based nanocomposites for electromagnetic wave absorption, EMI shielding, and photothermal conversion. Nano-Micro Letters. 2021 Dec;13(1):150.
18. Wu F, Zheng H, Wang W, Wu Q, Zhang Q, Guo J, Pu B, Shi X, Li J, Chen X, Hong W. Rapid eradication of antibiotic-resistant bacteria and biofilms by MXene and near-infrared Light through photothermal ablation. Science China Materials. 2021 Mar 1;64(3):748–58.
19. Zhou X, Wang Z, Chan YK, Yang Y, Jiao Z, Li L, Li J, Liang K, Deng Y. Infection micromilieu-activated nanocatalytic membrane for orchestrating rapid sterilization and stalled chronic wound regeneration. Advanced Functional Materials. 2022 Feb;32(7):2109469.
20. Rohaizad N, Mayorga-Martinez CC, Fojtů M, Latiff NM, Pumera M. Two-dimensional materials in biomedical, biosensing and sensing applications. Chemical Society Reviews. 2021;50(1):619–57.
21. Verma S, Dwivedi U, Chaturvedi K, Kumari N, Dhangar M, Hashmi SA, Singhal R, Srivastava AK. Progress of 2D MXenes based composites for efficient electromagnetic interference shielding applications: A review. Synthetic Metals. 2022 Jul 1;287:117095.
22. Tan C, Zhang H. Two-dimensional transition metal dichalcogenide nanosheet-based composites. Chemical Society Reviews. 2015;44(9):2713–31.
23. Gogotsi Y, Anasori B. The rise of MXenes. American Chemical Society Nano. 2019 Aug 27;13(8): 8491–4.
24. Singhwane A, Chaturvedi K, Mohapatra RK, Srivastava AK, Verma S. Mxene-based composite materials as antibacterial agents for healthcare applications. In Age of MXenes, Volume 2. Applications in Diagnostics, Therapeutics, and Environmental Remediation 2023. American Chemical Society, 2023, pp. 1–17.
25. Wyatt BC, Rosenkranz A, Anasori B. 2D MXenes: Tunable mechanical and tribological properties. Advanced Materials. 2021 Apr;33(17):2007973.
26. Huang Z, Cui X, Li S, Wei J, Li P, Wang Y, Lee C-S. Two-dimensional MXene-based materials for photothermal therapy. Nanophotonics. 2020;9. https://doi.org/10.1515/nanoph-2019-0571.
27. Alhabeb M, Maleski K, Anasori B, Lelyukh P, Clark L, Sin S, Gogotsi Y. Guidelines for synthesis and processing of two-dimensional titanium carbide ($Ti_3C_2T_x$ MXene). Chemistry of Materials. 2017;29:7633–7644.
28. Anasori B, Lukatskaya M, Gogotsi Y. 2D metal carbides and nitrides (MXenes) for energy storage. Nature Reviews Materials. 2017;2:16098. https://doi.org/10.1038/natrevmats.2016.98.
29. Hao, S., Han, H., Yang, Z. et al. Recent advancements on photothermal conversion and antibacterial applications over MXenes-based materials. Nano-Micro Letters. 2022;14:178. https://doi.org/10.1007/s40820-022-00901-w
30. Wu Z, Zhu S, Bai X, Liang M, Zhang X, Zhao N, He C. One-step in-situ synthesis of Sn-nanoconfined $Ti_3C_2T_x$ MXene composites for Li-ion battery anode. Electrochimica Acta. 2022 Mar 1;407:139916.
31. Koh SW, Rekhi L, Arramel, Birowosuto MD, Trinh QT, Ge J, Yu W, Wee AT, Choksi TS, Li H. Tuning the work function of MXene via surface functionalization. ACS Applied Materials & Interfaces. 2023 Dec 14;16 (49):66826–36.

32. Lin H, Chen Y, Shi J. Insights into 2D MXenes for versatile biomedical applications: Current advances and challenges ahead. Advanced Science. 2018 Oct;5(10):1800518.
33. Melancon MP, Zhou MI, Li C. Cancer theranostics with near-infrared light-activatable multimodal nanoparticles. Accounts of Chemical Research. 2011 Oct 18;44(10):947–56.
34. Yang K, Feng L, Shi X, Liu Z. Nano-graphene in biomedicine: theranostic applications. Chemical Society Reviews. 2013;42(2):530–47.
35. Sai DL, Lee J, Nguyen DL, Kim YP. Tailoring photosensitive ROS for advanced photodynamic therapy. Experimental & Molecular Medicine. 2021 Apr;53(4):495–504.
36. Okazaki T, Hirota N, Nagata T, Osuka A, Terazima M. High temporally and spatially resolved thermal energy detection after nonradiative transition in solution using a molecular heater– molecular thermometer integrated system. Journal of the American Chemical Society. 1999 May 14;121(21):5079–80.
37. Van der Zee J. Heating the patient: A promising approach?. Annals of oncology. 2002 Aug 1;13(8):1173–84.
38. Sharma, S., Batra, S., Chauhan, M.K., Kumar, V. (2023). Photothermal Therapy for Cancer Treatment. In Malviya, R., Sundram, S. (eds) Targeted Cancer Therapy in Biomedical Engineering. Biological and Medical Physics, Biomedical Engineering. Springer, Singapore. https://doi.org/10.1007/978-981-19-9786-0_22
39. Pattani, V.P., Shah, J., Atalis, A. et al. Role of apoptosis and necrosis in cell death induced by nanoparticle-mediated photothermal therapy. Journal of Nanoparticle Research. 2015;17:20. https://doi.org/10.1007/s11051-014-2822-3
40. Li H, Fan R, Zou B, Yan J, Shi Q, Guo G. Roles of MXenes in biomedical applications: Recent developments and prospects. Journal of Nanobiotechnology. 2023 Dec;21(1):1–39.
41. Lin H, Wang Y, Gao S, Chen Y, Shi J. Theranostic 2D tantalum carbide (MXene). Advanced Materials. 2018 Jan;30(4):1703284.
42. Wang D, Fang Y, Yu W, Wang L, Xie H, Yue Y. Significant solar energy absorption of MXene $Ti_3C_2T_x$ nanofluids via localized surface plasmon resonance. Solar Energy Materials and Solar Cells. 2021 Jan 1;220: 110850.
43. Xu D, Li Z, Li L, Wang J. Insights into the photothermal conversion of 2D MXene nanomaterials: Synthesis, mechanism, and applications. Advanced Functional Materials. 2020 Nov;30(47):2000712.
44. Tee SY, Win KY, Goh SS, Teng CP, Tang KY, Regulacio MD, Li Z, Ye E. Introduction to photothermal nanomaterials. Photothermal Nanomaterials. 2022 Jan 13;54:1.
45. Ye L, Cao Z, Liu X, Cui Z, Li Z, Liang Y, Zhu S, Wu S. Noble metal-based nanomaterials as antibacterial agents. Journal of Alloys and Compounds. 2022 May 25;904:164091.
46. Dediu V, Ghitman J, Gradisteanu Pircalabioru G, Chan KH, Iliescu FS, Iliescu C. Trends in photothermal nanostructures for antimicrobial applications. International Journal of Molecular Sciences. 2023 May 27;24(11):9375.
47. Tee SY, Win KY, Goh SS, Teng CP, Tang KY, Regulacio MD, ... Ye E., in E. Ye and Z. Li (eds.) Photothermal Nanomaterials. Introduction to Photothermal Nanomaterials. The Royal Society of Chemistry, 2022, ch. 1, pp. 1–32.

48. Shahzad F, Alhabeb M, Hatter CB, Anasori B, Man Hong S, Koo CM, Gogotsi Y. Electromagnetic interference shielding with 2D transition metal carbides (MXenes). Science. 2016 Sep 9;353(6304):1137–40. https://doi.org/10.1126/science.aag2421. PMID: 27609888.
49. Fan X, Liu L, Jin X, Wang W, Zhang S, Tang B. MXene $Ti_3C_2T_x$ for phase change composite with superior photothermal storage capability. Journal of Materials Chemistry A. 2019;7(23):14319–27.
50. Furube A, Hashimoto S. Insight into plasmonic hot-electron transfer and plasmon molecular drive: New dimensions in energy conversion and nanofabrication. NPG Asia Materials. 2017 Dec;9(12):e454.
51. Lipatov A, Alhabeb M, Lukatskaya MR, Boson A, Gogotsi Y, Sinitskii A. Effect of synthesis on quality, electronic properties and environmental stability of individual monolayer Ti_3C_2 MXene flakes. Advanced Electronic Materials. 2016 Dec;2(12):1600255.
52. Lin H, Wang X, Yu L, Chen Y, Shi J. Two-dimensional ultrathin MXene ceramic nanosheets for photothermal conversion. Nano Letters. 2017 Jan 11;17(1):384–391. https://doi.org/10.1021/acs.nanolett.6b04339. Epub 2016 Dec 30. PMID: 28026960.
53. Chaudhuri K, Alhabeb M, Wang Z, Shalaev VM, Gogotsi Y, Boltasseva A. Highly broadband absorber using plasmonic titanium carbide (MXene). ACS Photonics. 2018 Jan 10;5(3):1115–22.
54. Naguib M, Mochalin VN, Barsoum MW, Gogotsi Y. 25th anniversary article: MXenes: a new family of two-dimensional materials. Advanced Materials. 2014 Feb;26(7):992–1005.
55. Xiang Z, Shi Y, Zhu X, Cai L, Lu W. Flexible and waterproof 2D/1D/0D construction of MXene-based nanocomposites for electromagnetic wave absorption, EMI shielding, and photothermal conversion. Nano-Micro Letters. 2021 Dec;13(1):150.
56. Lin H, Gao S, Dai C, Chen Y, Shi J. A two-dimensional biodegradable niobium carbide (MXene) for photothermal tumor eradication in NIR-I and NIR-II biowindows. Journal of the American Chemical Society. 2017 Nov 15;139(45):16235–47.
57. Dai C, Chen Y, Jing X, Xiang L, Yang D, Lin H, Liu Z, Han X, Wu R. Two-dimensional tantalum carbide (MXenes) composite nanosheets for multiple imaging-guided photothermal tumor ablation. American Chemical Society Nano. 2017 Dec 26;11(12):12696–712.
58. Yu X, Cai X, Cui H, Lee SW, Yu XF, Liu B. Fluorine-free preparation of titanium carbide MXene quantum dots with high near-infrared photothermal performances for cancer therapy. Nanoscale. 2017;9(45):17859–64.
59. Shao J, Zhang J, Jiang C, Lin J, Huang P. Biodegradable titanium nitride MXene quantum dots for cancer phototheranostics in NIR-I/II biowindows. Chemical Engineering Journal. 2020 Nov 15;400:126009.
60. Rosenkranz A, Perini G, Aguilar-Hurtado JY, Zambrano DF, Wang B, Niccolini B, Henriques PC, Rosa E, De Maio F, Delogu G, De Spirito M. Laser-mediated antibacterial effects of few-and multi-layer Ti3C2Tx MXenes. Applied Surface Science. 2021 Nov 30;567:150795.
61. Wu F, Zheng H, Wang W, Wu Q, Zhang Q, Guo J, Pu B, Shi X, Li J, Chen X, Hong W. Rapid eradication of antibiotic-resistant bacteria and biofilms by

MXene and near-infrared Light through photothermal ablation. Science China Materials. 2021 Mar 1;64(3):748–58.
62. Zhu X, Zhu Y, Jia K, Abraha BS, Li Y, Peng W, Zhang F, Fan X, Zhang L. A near-infrared light-mediated antimicrobial based on Ag/$Ti_3C_2T_x$ for effective synergetic antibacterial applications. Nanoscale. 2020;12(37):19129–41.
63. Nie X, Wu S, Huang F, Li W, Qiao H, Wang Q, Wei Q. "Dew-of-Leaf" structure multiple synergetic antimicrobial modality hybrid: A rapid and long lasting bactericidal material. Chemical Engineering Journal. 2021 Jul 15;416:129072.
64. Li Q, Wang W, Feng H, Cao L, Wang H, Wang D, Chen S. NIR-triggered photocatalytic and photothermal performance for sterilization based on copper sulfide nanoparticles anchored on $Ti_3C_2T_x$ MXene. Journal of Colloid and Interface Science. 2021 Dec 15;604:810–22.
65. Jia Q, Song Q, Li P, Huang W. Rejuvenated photodynamic therapy for bacterial infections. Advanced healthcare materials. 2019 Jul;8(14):1900608.
66. Mosaddad SA, Namanloo RA, Aghili SS, Maskani P, Alam M, Abbasi K, Nouri F, Tahmasebi E, Yazdanian M, Tebyaniyan H. Photodynamic therapy in oral cancer: A review of clinical studies. Medical Oncology. 2023 Feb 7;40(3):91.
67. Sargazi S, Simge ER, Gelen SS, Rahdar A, Bilal M, Arshad R, Ajalli N, Khan MF, Pandey S. Application of titanium dioxide nanoparticles in photothermal and photodynamic therapy of cancer: An updated and comprehensive review. Journal of Drug Delivery Science and Technology. 2022 Jul 19;75(September 2022):103605.
68. Li X, Lovell JF, Yoon J, Chen X. Clinical development and potential of photothermal and photodynamic therapies for cancer. Nature Reviews Clinical Oncology. 2020 Nov;17(11):657–74.
69. Wang YY, Liu YC, Sun H, Guo DS. Type I photodynamic therapy by organic–inorganic hybrid materials: From strategies to applications. Coordination Chemistry Reviews. 2019 Sep 15;395:46–62.
70. Chen D, Xu Q, Wang W, Shao J, Huang W, Dong X. Type I photosensitizers revitalizing photodynamic oncotherapy. Small. 2021 Aug;17(31):2006742.
71. dos Santos AF, de Almeida DQ, Terra LF, Baptista MS, Labriola L. Photodynamic therapy in cancer treatment-an update review. Journal of Cancer Metastasis and Treatment. 2019 Mar 29;5(25):10–20517
72. Li X, Kwon N, Guo T, Liu Z, Yoon J. Innovative strategies for hypoxic-tumor photodynamic therapy. Angewandte Chemie International Edition. 2018 Sep 3;57(36):11522–31.
73. Naguib M, Kurtoglu M, Presser V, Lu J, Niu J, Heon M, Hultman L, Gogotsi Y, Barsoum MW. Two-dimensional nanocrystals produced by exfoliation of Ti_3AlC_2. Advanced Materials. 2011 Oct 4;23(37):4248–53.
74. Zhu B, Song P, Li J, Cao S, Shi J. Ti_3C_2 MXene/gold nanorods-based hybrid nanoparticles with photodynamic antibacterial activities. Journal of Materials Science. 2022 Nov;57(42):19957–71.
75. Feng H, Wang W, Wang T, Pu Y, Ma C, Chen S. Interfacial regulation of BiOI@ Bi_2S_3/MXene heterostructures for enhanced photothermal and photodynamic therapy in antibacterial applications. Acta Biomaterialia. 2023 Nov 1;171:506–18.

76. Wang J, Xuan J, Liu Y, Li Z, Han Y, Wang Z. NIR-dependent photothermal-photodynamic synergistic antibacterial mechanism for titanium carbide nanosheets intercalated and delaminated by tetramethylammonium hydroxide. Biomaterials Advances. 2023 Jun 6:213492.
77. Liu X, Xie H, Zhuo S, Zhou Y, Selim MS, Chen X, Hao Z. Ru(II) complex grafted $Ti_3C_2T_x$ MXene nano sheet with photothermal/photodynamic synergistic antibacterial activity. Nanomaterials. 2023;13:958. https://doi.org/10.3390/nano13060958.

5

Significance of MXene in Tissue Engineering: A Review

Manal M. Khan, Gaurav Chaturvedi, Ved Prakash Rao, and Madhuri Arora

5.1 Introduction

A significant public health concern is the lack of tissue and organs, as only a tiny proportion of worthy patients can get transplants [1,2]. Since only the sick seek aid like this, most waiting lists for tissues and organs fail to adequately reflect the severity of the problem [3–6]. In this review, the phrases 'tissue engineering' and 'regenerative medicine,' which often used interchangeably by researchers and physicians, are used. The possibility of repairing and replacing damaged tissues and organs is the cornerstone of regenerative medicine's promise. The field of regenerative medicine has delivered favorable results in the regeneration activity and replacement of several tissues and organs, incudes the liver, skin, kidney, and heart. It also holds promise for correcting some congenital disabilities [7,8].

The issues of donor scarcity and potential immune rejection of donated body parts confront the conventional dependence on donors for organs for transplantations [9,10]. Among the organ transplants carried out in poor countries are instances of 'transplant tourism,' in which wealthy and powerful foreigners are granted preference over the native population [11,12].

Since they may lead to exploiting helpless individuals, such techniques have been denounced [13,14]. Overcoming obstacles like the limited supply of organs and the logistical challenges associated with gathering them can help increase the number of people who can receive transplants, even in the face of variations in national economic powers and in the healthcare framework [15,16]. Thus, more work must be done on developing methods and tools to expand the availability of organs for transplantation. When people are injured in accidents or natural disasters, tissues and organs are typically needed immediately for transplantation [17].

The lack of tissues and organs makes medical care more complicated and scientific study more difficult. Therefore, the greatest challenge of our time is

DOI: 10.1201/9781003353287-5

to generate infinite tissues and organs. Numerous efforts have been made to improve organ use and promote organ donations [18–20]. The development of humanized animal organs, bioartificial organs, and laboratory-grown tissues is one option [21,22]. Some of these problems might be resolved using regenerative medicine [23,24].

3D printing is among the most remarkable technological developments of the past few decades [25]. The most significant advancement has been the uninterrupted printing of biomaterial onto a scaffold for potential cell seeding, a process known as 3D bioprinting. This technique demands multiple disciplines, which include tissue engineering, material science, and cell biology. The exact placement of biological components, cells, and biomolecules like growth factors is necessary for successful bioprinting. 3D bioprinting needs to accurately reproduce the complex architecture of the ECM (extracellular matrix) and the variety of cells present in different tissues in order to adequately simulate human tissue. Additionally, the circulatory and neurological systems of each required tissue must be recapitulated by bioprinting [26,27].

In this chapter, we discuss the latest developments and the successful implementation of tissue engineering approaches in skin regeneration, bone repair, cartilage restoration, and organ transplantation. Additionally, MXenes and their significance in tissue engineering are reviewed herein. MXenes' special features—such as their biocompatibility, mechanical strength, and high conductivity—make them attractive options for enhancing the performance of biomaterials in tissue engineering fields.

5.2 Tissue Engineering: A Concise Overview

The discipline of tissue engineering is multidisciplinary, utilizing concepts from material science, biology, and engineering to produce 3D, functional organs. Tissue engineering's main concept is to enhance patients' quality of life by creating means of replacing or mending diseased or damaged tissues. Biomaterials are essential to tissue engineering because they act as scaffolds, transporters, or matrices for cells to adhere, multiply, and differentiate [28,29].

Important elements of using biomaterials in tissue engineering comprise:

1. **Biomaterials:** Materials designed specifically to work with biological systems to replace or mend tissues are known as biomaterials.
    - They may be synthetic, natural, or a mix.
    - Composite materials, metals, ceramics, and polymers are a few examples.

2. **Scaffolds:** Scaffolds are three-dimensional components that offer a structure for the attachment, growth, and development of cells into tissues.
   - They function as a mechanical scaffolding and tissue development guide, emulating the extracellular matrix.
   - Scaffolds that decompose naturally are frequently employed so that the newly created tissue can gradually replace them.
3. **Cells:** Because they are responsible for creating functional tissue, cells are essential to tissue engineering.
   - Because they may differentiate into numerous cell types, stem cells—including pluripotent and adult stem cells—are frequently used in medical applications.
4. **Growth factors:** Signaling molecules known as growth factors control cell behavior and promote tissue regeneration. They can be given independently or integrated with biomaterials to improve tissue development.
5. **Bioreactors:** Bioreactors are apparatuses used to produce a regulated environment for in vitro tissue growth. They mimic physiological

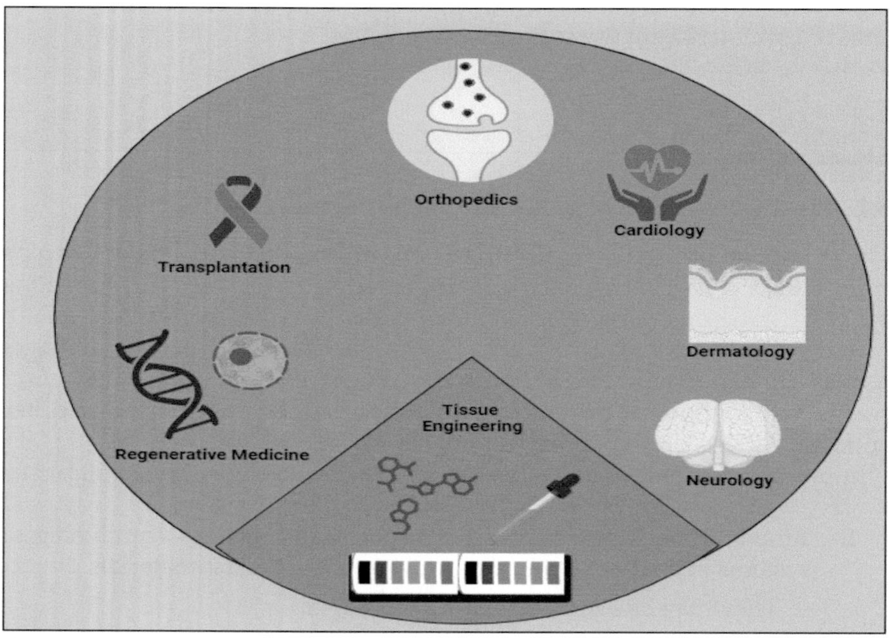

FIGURE 5.1
Tissue engineering applications across diverse fields.

circumstances by supplying nutrients, removing waste, and providing mechanical stimulation.

Medical outlook:
Tissue engineering has promising implementations in various medical fields as illustrated in Figure 5.1.

While tissue engineering with biomaterials has made significant strides, challenges remain, including achieving vascularization in ensuring long-term functionality, engineered tissues, and highlighting the immunological concerns. Continued study and research advancements in the field are necessary to realize the full potential of tissue engineering in clinical applications.

5.3 Advancing Health Care Through Tissue Engineering: A Comprehensive Exploration

In the collaborative pursuit of groundbreaking healthcare solutions, various researchers have explored tissue engineering comprehensively. This collaborative endeavor delves into the intricate world of tissue regeneration, focusing on addressing injuries, congenital disabilities, and degenerative diseases. The interdisciplinary nature of this research, undertaken by experts from diverse fields, propels the field forward, offering a glimpse into a future where tissue engineering is pivotal in advancing healthcare outcomes. Through this concerted exploration, researchers strive to unlock the full potential of tissue engineering, paving the way for transformative applications in regenerative medicine and organ transplantation.

Yoshio Hori and his colleagues [30] set out to study in 2002 how the induction of the muscular layer was affected by the seeding of mesenchymal stem cells (MSCs) onto the collagen scaffold, as shown in Figure 5.2. They used beagle dogs in an animal experiment to examine the impact of the scaffold regarding muscle layer regeneration by MSC seeding. According to the outcome, they were able to successfully regenerate the small intestine by tissue engineering methods. Nevertheless, it was discovered that the regenerated gut lacked the muscle layer necessary for normal peristalsis. We concentrated on using autologous MSC as a resource for tissue of muscle to promote regeneration of the muscular layer.

In this work, Sato et al. 2003 [31] performed an allografting method to regenerate the injured AF and NP using tissue-engineering techniques. After laser vaporizing the NP of rabbit intervertebral discs, they introduced AF fibroblasts cultured within the ACHMS scaffold inside the disc cavity. Restoring the functionality of intervertebral disc tissue is as crucial as restoring its anatomic shape. The outcomes demonstrated the proliferative activity and viability of the allografted AF cells in vivo. These first findings indicate that

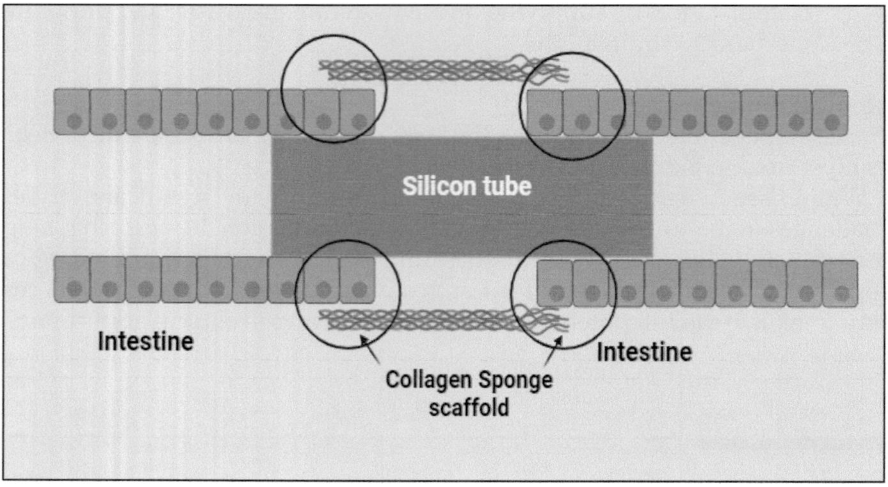

FIGURE 5.2
Systematic presentation of the operative procedure.

intervertebral disc regeneration may be achievable by allografting AF cells, despite some issues still needing to be resolved.

Using this experiment, Ralf Sodian et al. [32] assessed whether scaffold material and in vitro conditioning were suitable for producing viable tissue for trileaflet heart valve tissue engineering. They constructed a trileaflet heart valve scaffold that is elastic and porous using a biodegradable polymer called polyhydroxyalkanoate. Vascular cells were seeded onto the scaffold and exposed to pulsatile flow to allow the polymer to combine with the cells. The manufactured cardiac valve scaffolds appeared malleable and functioned appropriately in supraphysiologic and subphysiologic flow settings. The purpose of using a porous, three-dimensional polymer was to enhance the polymer's surface area, allowing for more cells to attach to the heart valve scaffold.

The findings showed that when cells were deposited onto a porous PHA scaffold connected to this polymer, they produced a confluent and orientated cell layer following exposure to pulsatile flow. Furthermore, under in vitro pulsatile flow circumstances, the results have shown the ability to produce collagen as assessed by the hydroxyproline test and glycosaminoglycans as stained by the movant, as well as the proliferation of vascular cells (DNA assay). The tissue-engineered structures' absence of elastin may be one of this method's drawbacks. Consequently, more research is required to advance our in vitro methods for producing an extracellular matrix that fully resembles natural vascular tissue. Another noteworthy finding from this experiment was that the cells moved into pores and created tissue bridges connecting the interior and exterior.

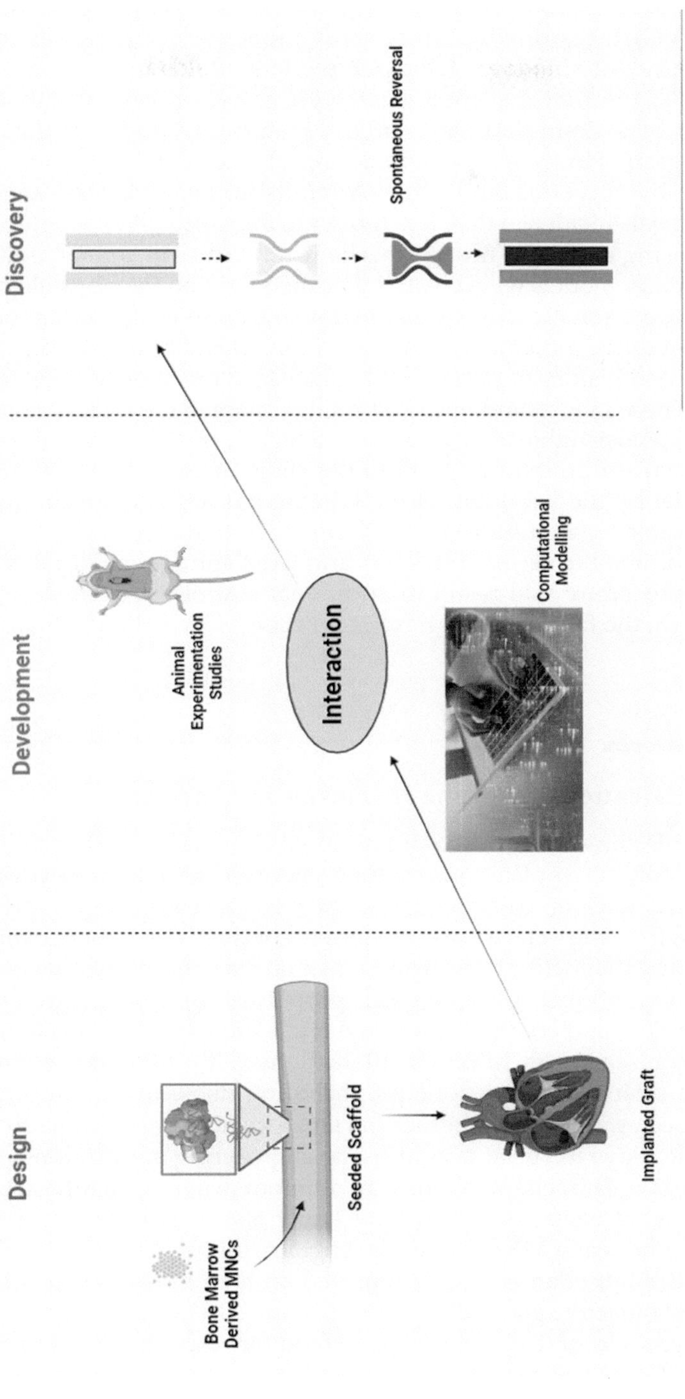

FIGURE 5.3
A tissue-engineered vascular graft (TEVG).

In 2023, Breuer and his colleagues created a tissue-engineered vasculature graft (TEVG) by sprinkling autologous mononuclear cells obtained from bone marrow into biodegradable polymeric scaffolds in the shape of tubes. This TEVG, the first designed graft with growth potential, demonstrated feasibility in a first-in-human study, transforming into a living, growing vascular graft. However, the initial clinical research, evaluating safety as approved by the Food and Drug Administration, indicated a premature TEVG stenosis incidence that was too high, impeding the widespread use of this promising method. Through mechanistic studies in animal models, complex computer models were created that shed light on the physiology of stenosis. Computational models demonstrated a distinct inflammation-driven, mechano-mediated method for in vivo TEVG development and revealed an unanticipated history of nature, which included the spontaneous reversal of stenosis. These in vivo and in silico findings enabled the logical development of TEVG stenosis inhibition strategies, which were confirmed in preclinical large animal studies and brought to the clinic through a recently approved clinical trial by the Food and Drug Administration. This breakthrough was made possible by a multidisciplinary approach that included computational simulations and the use of both small and large animal models. It is expected that this procedure will result in additional scaffold pattern developments and, in turn, the fabrication of next-generation TEVGs (Figure 5.3).

5.4 Significance of MXene in Tissue Engineering

Recently, MXene—a novel two-dimensional (2D) material—has drawn much attention. MXene applications include energy conversion, electromagnetic interference, sensors, electrochemical storage capacitors, and catalysts [34]. Because of their high electrical and thermal conductivity, superior mechanical qualities, and distinctive optical and plasmon features, planar nanostructures and the exceptional physiological properties of micro-supercapacitors, power sources, and energy collection devices are advantageous to them [35]. Moreover, research on MXene's interactions with biological elements has shown its biological characteristics, including its ability to induce reactive oxygen species, convert photothermal energy, and have antimicrobial effects [36]. It also plays a crucial part in tissue engineering applications, as shown in Figure 5.4. This chapter looks at different ways to synthesize MXene, discusses what researchers currently know about its biological properties, and looks into using MXene in tissue engineering.

The research by Pan et al. [37] reported on the innovative combination of 3D-printed bioactive glass (BG) scaffolds with 2D Ti_3C_2 MXene (referred to as Ti_3C_2-BG scaffold or TBGS) to achieve simultaneous photonic hyperthermia

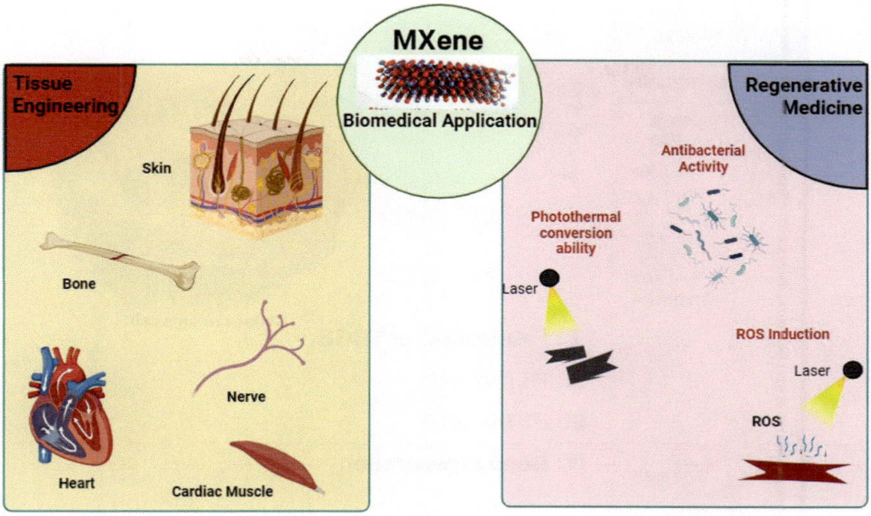

FIGURE 5.4
Biomedical applications of MXene in tissue engineering and regenerative medicines.

to ablate bone tumors and bioactive scaffolds to regenerate bone tissue, as illustrated in Figure 5.5. The developed composite scaffolds cause bone tumor ablation by near-infrared-triggered photothermal hyperthermia, which results in the total removal of tumors in vivo on bone-tumor xenografts. This is achieved by utilizing the exceptionally high photothermal transformation efficiency of 2D Ti_3C_2 MXene. Crucially, the deliberate addition of 2D MXene Ti_3C_2 greatly quickens the process by which newborn bone tissue forms in vivo inside the assembled BG scaffolds. The Ti_3C_2 MXene-integrated composite scaffolds show significant promise for treating bone tumors due to their dual capacity to kill the tumors and regenerate bone tissue. This greatly expands the biomedical potential of 2D MXenes in tissue engineering.

In a 2022 study by Mi and coworkers [38], they fabricated a composite scaffold consisting of HA and SA that was modified with Ti_3C_2-MXene and created via extrusion-stationed 3D printing. This is the only work that has utilized extrusion-based 3D printing to construct Ti_3C_2-modified sodium alginate and hydroxyapatite (HA/SA) composite scaffolds. BMSCs were utilized in the in vitro osteogenic potential and biocompatibility studies of the scaffolds. Additionally, to study the scaffold's impact on in vivo bone regeneration, a model was developed—a critical-sized rat calvarial bone lesion. The outcomes demonstrated the great mechanical strength, consistent structure, and macropore shape of the produced scaffold. The scaffold demonstrated remarkable biocompatibility with BMSCs, facilitated cell proliferation, and elevated alkaline phosphatase activity along with osteogenic gene expression.

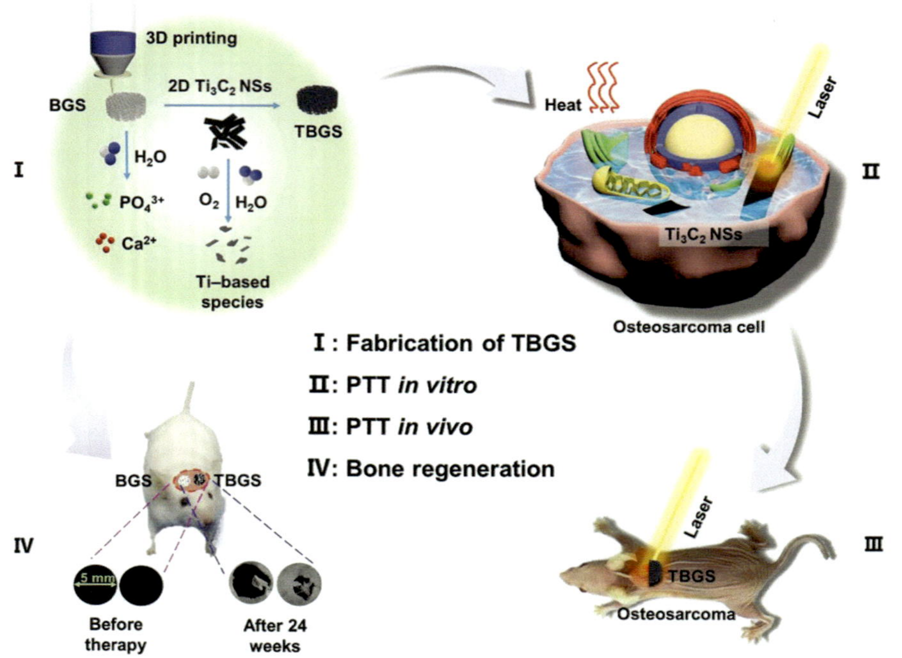

FIGURE 5.5
TBGS fabrication, bone cancer is abated, and bone tissue regenerates. (I) The TBGS fabrication process, which includes the combination of MXene Ti_3C_2, the devastation of MXene Ti_3C_2 on BGS, and the 3D printing of pure BGS. (II, III) TBGS was utilized for in vitro (II) and in vivo (III) photothermal ablation-based osteosarcoma cell eradication. (IV) Bone tissue repair and therapeutic outcomes following BGS and TBGS implantation [37].

The results of the experiment demonstrated that the scaffold considerably outperformed scaffolds without additional Ti_3C_2 MXene in terms of bone healing and effectively enhanced bone regeneration in an instance of critical-size calvarial bone defect in vivo. In summary, the 3D-printed scaffolds made from Ti_3C_2 MXene composites demonstrate significant potential for treating clinical bone defects. The results of this investigation offer a theoretical foundation for creating realistic uses for tissue-engineered bone scaffolds.

In their work, Diedkova et al. [39] developed biocompatible and biodegradable nanofiber scaffolds through electrospinning polycaprolactone (PCL), as shown in Figure 5.6. To clarify the deporosity of nanofiber scaffolds and defective pattern, they immobilized Ti_3C_2Tx MXene in numerous coatings on the electrically spun PCL membrane and combined additional techniques with positron annihilation experiments. The polymer base was characterized by the presence of nanopores. A voltage resonance at 8 × 104 Hz with a relaxed duration of 6.5 × 106 s was discovered in the

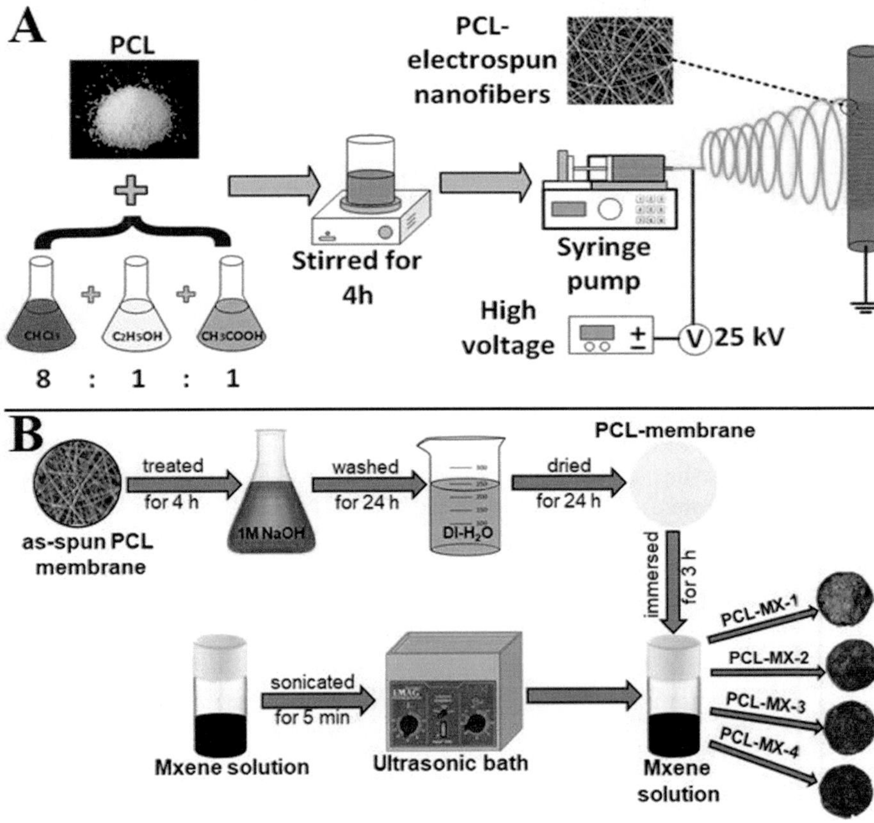

FIGURE 5.6
Principal scheme of the electrospinning process that was used to obtain PCL [36].

20–355 K temperature interval. The MXene surface layers exhibited a large abundance of vacancies at temperatures between 305 and 355 K. Based on the annealing temperature, a long-lived element of the positron lifespan emerged. The potential application of MXene-coated PCL membranes as a conductive biomaterial was demonstrated by investigating the composite scaffolds' conductivity throughout a broad temperature parameter, indulging its inductive and capacity components. In vitro testing and bacterial tests revealed a correlation between the electrical structure of MXene, the faults that developed in its layers, and the biological characteristics of the scaffolds. With modest antibacterial properties, double and triple MXene coatings created a favorable cell adhesion and growth environment. The PCL–MXene composite's structural, chemical, electrical, and biological characteristics showed its superiority over the current conductive scaffolds for tissue engineering.

In 2023, Shilei Li and colleagues [40] proposed the use of microstructure Ti-6Al-4V scaffolds with a diamond-like quality for customized bone defect healing. These scaffolds aim to mimic the mechanical characteristics of native bone tissue while fostering bone ingrowth and integration. Several coats of Ti_3C_2Tx/HAp assembled coverings were produced onto the contoured surface within 3D-printed porous scaffolds utilizing the pulsed electrodeposition process in order to prepare various biological functional coatings. Delaminated Ti_3C_2Tx has been studied using transmission electron microscopy (TEM), which shows an incredibly thin microstructure that is evenly distributed throughout the electrolyte. Characterization via X-ray diffraction (XRD) provides evidence for this.

Scanning electron microscopy shows a high association between the concentration of Ti_3C_2Tx and the morphology of composite coatings because efficient voltages for electrodeposition are available. The results of testing utilizing linear scanning voltammetry and electrochemical impedance spectroscopy show that the Ti_3C_2Tx/HAp constructed covering has the best corrosion resistance. To verify the Ti_3C_2Tx/HAp coating's resistance to corrosion in a physiological setting, the coating's in vitro electrolytic deterioration was examined using human-simulated bodily fluid. Using in vitro MC3T3-E1 cell cultivation experiments, the cell behaviors and biocompatibility of coatings were evaluated. The results show that cells grow on the outermost layer of composite coatings healthily without displaying cytotoxicity, and that their morphologies show a growing inward orientation and a good spreading condition.

To stop cancer recurrence and encourage bone formation, Zhang et al. [41] devised a unique multifunctional scaffold material composed mainly of g-C_3N_4, MXene nanosheets, and nano-hydroxyapatite particles (n-HA). The scaffolds exhibit both photothermal and photodynamic effects simultaneously under NIR irradiation thanks to the integration of g-C_3N_4 and MXene, and the proliferation of osteosarcoma cells is inhibited by N-HA. Remarkably, at 45°C, n-HA may augment the synergistic antitumor characteristics of photodynamic as well as photothermal techniques, and the scaffolds may eliminate osteosarcoma cells in about 10 minutes. The scaffold can also promote osteogenic growth in the bone marrow mesenchymal cell lines and is highly cytocompatible. Therefore, employing NIR irradiation, this adaptable scaffold may quickly stop bone tumors, prevent the growth of bone tumor cells, and promote osteogenic activity. Following the removal of a bone malignancy, tissue damage may be addressed with this potential technique.

Rui Luo et al.'s work from 2023 [42] shows how PTT and a scaffold for tissue engineering make sense together to create the Ti_3C_2 MXene, silk, fibroin, collagen, with quercetin composite scaffold (M-CSQ scaffold), which is shown in Figure 5.7. This biomaterial, which can be 3D printed, can both kill oral squamous cell carcinoma (OSCC) cells and encourage the healing of mucosal defects. The M-CSQ scaffolds contain enough porosity to permit adequate

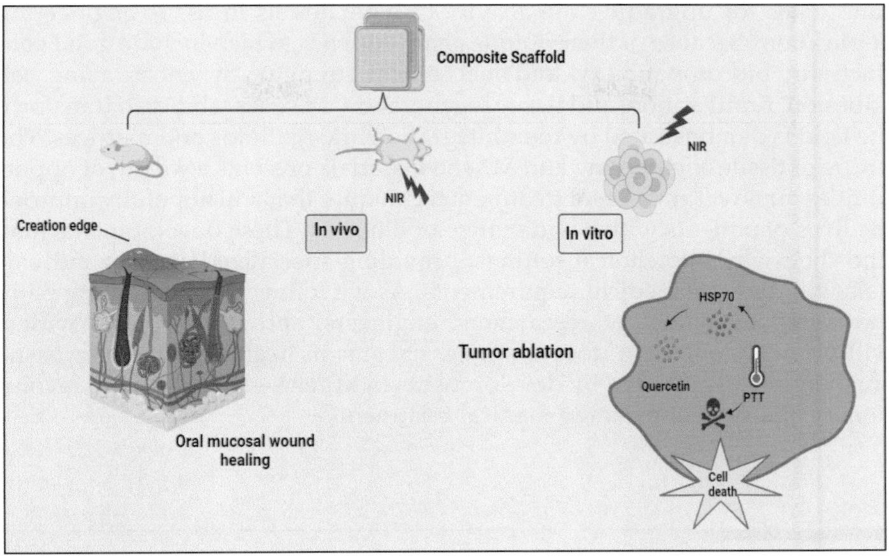

FIGURE 5.7
The formation of composite scaffold (M-CSQ scaffold).

cell movement and serve as a proliferative zone. They were developed using cryo 3D printing and freezing and drying processes. Remarkable durability and photothermal conversion characteristics are displayed by Ti_3C_2 MXene. Because quercetin decreased HSP70 expression, OSCC cells were less able to tolerate high temperatures, which increased the effects of PTT.

The M-CSQ scaffold effectively inhibited the growth of tumors in vivo and killed OSCC cells in vitro. Additionally, M-CSQ scaffold and (SD rat) buccal mucosal cell adhesion sites promote the healing of buccal mucosal wounds.

5.5 Conclusion and Future Perspectives

In summary, the astounding developments in tissue engineering signify a revolutionary new direction in medical research that has the potential to change the face of health care completely. The field has advanced toward novel approaches to tissue regeneration and repair through biomaterials, complex scaffolds, and cellular methods. Globally, scientists have worked together to push the frontiers of understanding, tackle important issues, and get regenerative medicine one step closer to real-world applications. Furthermore, tissue engineering now has a new dimension thanks to the noteworthy emergence of the two-dimensional nanomaterial MXene. MXenes are promising candidates for upgrading the activity of biomaterials in tissue engineering applications because of their unique characteristics, which include good conductivity, biocompatibility, and mechanical strength. By encouraging cell adhesion, proliferation, and tissue regeneration, MXenes' ability to transform the field is demonstrated by their integration into scaffolds and matrices. The future of tissue engineering and MXene materials presents a wealth of opportunities for novel and potent treatment techniques that will hopefully improve the lives of patients with a wide range of illnesses. These developments may find their way into clinical settings, providing specialized care for individuals with various medical requirements. As we follow this fascinating path, the combined efforts of researchers, engineers, and healthcare providers will probably open the door to a new chapter in healthcare history: tissue engineering—supported by developments in MXene—contributes to revolutionary and patient-centered medical treatments.

References

1. K. Dzobo, N. E. Thomford, D. A. Senthebane, H. Shipanga, A. Rowe, C. Dandara, M. Pillay, and K. S. C. M. Motaung, "Advances in regenerative medicine and tissue engineering: Innovation and transformation of medicine," Stem Cells International, vol. 2018, pp. 1–24, 2018. https://doi.org/10.1155/2018/2495848.
2. B. Jones and M. Bes, "Keeping kidneys," Bulletin of the World Health Organization, vol. 90, no. 10, pp. 718–719, 2012.
3. M. Colvin, J. M. Smith, M. A. Skeans et al., "OPTN/SRTR 2015 annual data report: Heart," American Journal of Transplantation, vol. 17, Supplement 1, pp. 286–356, 2017.
4. A. Hart, J. M. Smith, M. A. Skeans et al., "OPTN/SRTR 2015 annual data report: Kidney," American Journal of Transplantation, vol. 17, Supplement 1, pp. 21–116, 2017.
5. A. K. Israni, D. Zaun, C. Bolch et al., "OPTN/SRTR 2015 annual data report: Deceased organ donation," American Journal of Transplantation, vol. 17, Supplement 1, pp. 503–542, 2017.
6. B. L. Kasiske, S. K. Asrani, M. A. Dew et al., "The living donor collective: A scientific registry for living donors," American Journal of Transplantation, vol. 17, no. 12, pp. 3040–3048, 2017.
7. S. Nagral, M. Hussain, S. A. Nayeem, R. Dias, S. A. Enam, and S. Nundy, "Unmet need for surgery in south Asia," BMJ, vol. 357, article j1423, 2017.
8. H. C. Ott, T. S. Matthiesen, S. K. Goh et al., "Perfusion-decellularized matrix: Using nature's platform to engineer a bioartificial heart," Nature Medicine, vol. 14, no. 2, pp. 213–221, 2008.
9. D. J. Lo, B. Kaplan, and A. D. Kirk, "Biomarkers for kidney transplant rejection," Nature Reviews Nephrology, vol. 10, no. 4, pp. 215–225, 2014.

10. K. J. Wood and R. Goto, "Mechanisms of rejection: Current perspectives," Transplantation, vol. 93, no. 1, pp. 1–10, 2012.
11. J. R. Chapman, "Seeking to close the loopholes in transplant tourism and organ trafficking," Transplantation, vol. 102, no. 1, pp. 11–12, 2018.
12. J. J. O. Mogaka, L. Mupara, and J. M. Tsoka-Gwegweni, "Ethical issues associated with medical tourism in Africa," Journal of Market Access & Health Policy, vol. 5, no. 1, article 1309770, 2017.
13. Steering Committee of the Istanbul Summit, "Organ trafficking and transplant tourism and commercialism: The declaration of Istanbul," The Lancet, vol. 372, no. 9632, pp. 5–6, 2008.
14. International Summit on Transplant Tourism and Organ Trafficking, "The declaration of Istanbul on organ trafficking and transplant tourism," Saudi Journal of Kidney Diseases and Transplantation, vol. 21, no. 1, pp. 138–147, 2010.
15. R. W. Evans, D. L. Manninen, L. P. Garrison Jr, and A. M. Maier, "Donor availability as the primary determinant of the future of heart transplantation," JAMA: The Journal of the American Medical Association, vol. 255, no. 14, pp. 1892–1898, 1986.
16. D. L. Manninen and R. W. Evans, "Public attitudes and behavior regarding organ donation," JAMA: The Journal of the American Medical Association, vol. 253, no. 21, pp. 3111–3115, 1985.
17. J. Gill, C. Rose, J. Lesage, Y. Joffres, J. Gill, and K. O'Connor, "Use and outcomes of kidneys from donation after circulatory death donors in the United States," Journal of the American Society of Nephrology, vol. 28, no. 12, pp. 3647–3657, 2017.
18. S. Resnick, M. J. Seamon, D. Holena, J. Pascual, P. M. Reilly, and N. D. Martin, "Early declaration of death by neurologic criteria results in greater organ donor potential," Journal of Surgical Research, vol. 218, pp. 29–34, 2017.
19. M. Collin, J. Karpelowsky, and G. Thomas, "Pediatric transplantation: An international perspective," Seminars in Pediatric Surgery, vol. 26, no. 4, pp. 272–277, 2017.
20. S. A. Hosgood and M. L. Nicholson, "The evolution of donation after circulatory death donor kidney repair in the United Kingdom," Current Opinion in Organ Transplantation, vol. 23, no. 1, pp. 130–135, 2017.
21. U. Maggiore, R. Oberbauer, J. Pascual et al., "Strategies to increase the donor pool and access to kidney transplantation: An international perspective," Nephrology Dialysis Transplantation, vol. 30, no. 2, pp. 217–222, 2015.
22. M. G. Francipane and E. Lagasse, "Toward organs on demand: Breakthroughs and challenges in models of organogenesis," Current Pathobiology Reports, vol. 4, no. 3, pp. 77–85, 2016.
23. A. Shafiee and A. Atala, "Tissue engineering: Toward a new era of medicine," Annual Review of Medicine, vol. 68, no. 1, pp. 29–40, 2017.
24. G. Orlando, P. di Cocco, M. D'Angelo, K. Clemente, A. Famulari, and F. Pisani, "Regenerative medicine applied to solid organ transplantation: Where do we stand?," Transplantation Proceedings, vol. 42, no. 4, pp. 1011–1013, 2010.
25. R. Pareta, B. Sanders, P. Babbar et al., "Immunoisolation: Where regenerative medicine meets solid organ transplantation," Expert Review of Clinical Immunology, vol. 8, no. 7, pp. 685–692, 2012.

26. A. V. Do, B. Khorsand, S. M. Geary, and A. K. Salem, "3D printing of scaffolds for tissue regeneration applications," Advanced Healthcare Materials, vol. 4, no. 12, pp. 1742–1762, 2015.
27. S. V. Murphy and A. Atala, "3D bioprinting of tissues and organs," Nature Biotechnology, vol. 32, no. 8, pp. 773–785, 2014.
28. Lanza, R., Langer, R., Vacanti, J. P. and Atala, A. eds., 2020. Principles of tissue engineering. Academic Press.
29. Palsson, B., Hubbell, J. A., Plonsey, R. and Bronzino, J. D. eds., 2003. Tissue engineering. CRC Press.
30. Y. Hori, T. Nakamura, D. Kimura, K. Kaino, Y. Kurokawa, S. Satomi, and Y. Shimizu, "Experimental study on tissue engineering of the small intestine by mesenchymal stem cell seeding," Journal of Surgical Research, vol. 102, no. 2, pp. 0–160, 2002. https://doi.org/10.1006/jsre.2001.6294.
31. M. Sato, T. Asazuma, M. Ishihara, M. Ishihara, T. Kikuchi, M. Kikuchi, K. Fujikawa, "An experimental study of the regeneration of the intervertebral disc with an allograft of cultured annulus fibrosus cells using a tissue-engineering method," Spine, vol. 28, no. 6, pp. 548–553, March 15, 2003. https://doi.org/10.1097/01.BRS.0000049909.09102.60.
32. R. Sodian, S. P. Hoerstrup, J. S. Sperling, S. H. Daebritz, D. P. Martin, F. J. Schoen, J. P. Vacanti, J. E. Mayer Jr, "Tissue engineering of heart valves: In vitro experiences," Annals of Thoracic Surgery, vol. 70, no. 1, 0–144, 2000. https://doi.org/10.1016/s0003-4975(00)01255-8.
33. T. Breuer, M. Jimenez, J. D. Humphrey, T. Shinoka, and C. K. Breuer, "Tissue engineering of vascular grafts: A case report from bench to bedside and back," Arteriosclerosis, Thrombosis, and Vascular Biology, vol. 43, no. 3, pp. 399–409, 2023. https://doi.org/10.1161/ATVBAHA.122.318236.
34. K. Chaturvedi, V. Hada, S. Paul, B. Sarma, D. Malvi, M. Dhangar, H. Bajpai, A. Singhwane, A. K. Srivastava, and S. Verma, "The rise of MXene: A Wonder 2D material, from its synthesis and properties to its versatile applications—A comprehensive review," Topics in Current Chemistry, vol. 381, no. 2, p. 11, 2023.
35. S. Verma, M. Dhangar, S. Paul, K. Chaturvedi, M. A. Khan, and A. K. Srivastava, "Recent advances for fabricating smart electromagnetic interference shielding textile: A comprehensive review," Electronic Materials Letters, vol. 18, no. 4, pp. 331–44, 2022.
36. A. Singhwane, K. Chaturvedi, R. K. Mohapatra, A. K. Srivastava, and S. Verma, Mxene-based composite materials as antibacterial agents for healthcare applications. In Age of MXenes, Volume 2. Applications in Diagnostics, Therapeutics, and Environmental Remediation 2023. American Chemical Society, 2023, pp. 1–17.
37. S. Pan, J. Yin, L. Yu, C. Zhang, Y. Zhu, Y. Gao, and Y. Chen, "2D MXene-integrated 3D-printing scaffolds for augmented osteosarcoma phototherapy and accelerated tissue reconstruction," Advanced Science, vol. 7, no. 2, p. 1901511, 2020.
38. X. Mi, Z. Su, Y. Fu, S. Li, and A. Mo, "3D printing of Ti3C2-MXene-incorporated composite scaffolds for accelerated bone regeneration," Biomedical Materials, vol. 17, no. 3, p. 035002, 2022.

39. K. Diedkova, A. D. Pogrebnjak, S. Kyrylenko, K. Smyrnova, V. V. Buranich, P. Horodek, P. Zukowski, T. N. Koltunowicz, P. Galaszkiewicz, K. Makashina, V. Bondariev, M. Sahul, M. Čaplovičová, Y. Husak, W. Simka, V. Korniienko, A. Stolarczyk, A. Blacha-Grzechnik, V. Balitskyi, V. Zahorodna, I. Baginskiy, U. Riekstina, O. Gogotsi, Y. Gogotsi, and M. Pogorielov, "Polycaprolactone–MXene nanofibrous scaffolds for tissue engineering," ACS Applied Materials & Interfaces, vol. 15, no. 11, pp. 14033–14047, 2023. https://doi.org/10.1021/acsami.2c22780.
40. S. Li, H. Lei, H. Liu, P. Song, S. Fan, L. Wu, D. Liao, G. Xian, L. Xiong, C. Zhou, and H. Fan, "Pulsed electrodeposition of MXenes/HAp multiple biological functional coatings on 3D printed porous Ti-6Al-4V bone tissue engineering scaffold," Surface and Coatings Technology, vol. 464, article no. 129532, 2023, ISSN 0257–8972, https://doi.org/10.1016/j.surfcoat.2023.129532.
41. G. Zhang, Y. Lu, J. Song, D. Huang, M. An, W. Chen, P. Han, X. Yao, and X. Zhang, "A multifunctional nano-hydroxyapatite/MXene scaffold for the photothermal/dynamic treatment of bone tumours and simultaneous tissue regeneration," Journal of Colloid and Interface Science, vol. 652, Part B, pp. 1673–1684, 2023, ISSN 0021-9797, https://doi.org/10.1016/j.jcis.2023.08.176.
42. R. Luo, F. Li, Y. Wang, H. Zou, J. Shang, Y. Fan, H. Liu, Z. Xu, R. Li, and H. Liu, "MXene-modified 3D printed scaffold for photothermal therapy and facilitation of oral mucosal wound reconstruction," Materials & Design, vol. 227, article no. 111731, 2023, ISSN 0264-1275, https://doi.org/10.1016/j.matdes.2023.111731.

6

MXene Marvels: Exploring the Insights and Applications of MXene-Based Materials in Wearable Technology for Healthcare Systems

Kamna Chaturvedi, Neelam Kumari, Umesh Dwivedi, and Sarika Verma

6.1 Introduction

The global healthcare framework is undergoing a rapid evolution that includes personalized health care, monitoring patients remotely, point-of-care medical diagnosis, and the medical Internet of Things. There has been a significant upsurge in wearable device research and commercialization [1,2]. Nonetheless, there have been advancements and disappointments in the creation of wearable sensors of a commercial caliber. The most recent developments in nanotechnology, downsizing, flexible electronics, wireless sensing technologies, and embedded systems open the door to the creation of intelligent platforms that offer personalized health monitoring regularly [3,4]. To continually and closely monitor health, soft wearable sensors are devices crafted for attachment directly onto the skin, conforming naturally to the body's structure. In this regard, laboratory-made epidermal electronic devices are being developed for clinical diagnosis of skin temperature, electromyography, respiration rate, heart rate, and sweating [5–9]. Biocompatible and biodegradable electronics can be used to treat a variety of ailments in addition to being able to clinically monitor a patient's health in the contours of smart wearable and implanted gadgets. In a similar vein, several research teams have created wearable technology that uses sensors based on tattoos and textiles which provide precise in situ metrics to track accurate data of different metabolites and electrolytes in a non-invasive manner. Still, the majority of wearables use sensing methods that are 10 years old. Transdermal glucose monitors, for instance, rely on

 DOI: 10.1201/9781003353287-6

inexpensive fingerprick test strips as their enzyme electrodes. Indeed, the transdermal glucose-sensing gadgets may be the most widely used wearable sensors which also track the progression of the underlying illness and objectively detect blood glucose concentration. Epidermal sensors' potential diagnostic capabilities might be discerned by resolving important manufacturing technological challenges and establishing a reliable correlation to standard sensing modalities [10].

In recent years, the rapid advancement of wearable technology has revolutionized various aspects of our lives, ranging from healthcare monitoring to fitness tracking and beyond. These devices, seamlessly integrated into our daily routines, have become indispensable tools for enhancing human performance, well-being, and connectivity. The demand for wearable technology that is lightweight, flexible, and durable has led to the exploration of novel materials. Among the diverse array of materials investigated for wearable device applications, MXenes have emerged as a particularly promising class of materials, for their unique combination of properties and versatile functionalities [11]. MXenes, a family of 2D transition metal carbides, nitrides, and carbonitrides, derived from layered MAX phases, offer an intriguing platform for the design and fabrication of wearable electronics [12]. Their exceptional electrical conductivity, mechanical strength, large surface area, and chemical stability make them well-suited for a broad range of wearable device areas.

This chapter provides a comprehensive overview of MXene-based materials for wearable devices in the healthcare system. To start with the key properties of MXene for wearable technology, a brief overview of the fabrication of sensing layers is also discussed. The chapter gives an idea about physical sensors and chemical sensors. Physical sensors include those sensors that contribute to pulse monitoring and human health activities monitoring such as facial expressions, voice recognition, and motion and gesture sensing. Chemical sensors include the electrochemical sensors used for sweat analysis and gas sensors.

Even though MXenes has bright futures in wearable technology, there are still several issues that need to be resolved. Several challenges stand in the way of their broad adoption, including biocompatibility, synthesis scalability, stability in physiological circumstances, and integration onto flexible substrates. To fully realize the potential of MXenes in this quickly developing sector, the chapter ends by describing future directions and research opportunities in the field of MXene-based wearable devices. It emphasizes the importance of interdisciplinary collaboration and ongoing innovation. MXenes are well-positioned to contribute significantly to the development of wearable technology by providing customized, linked, and seamlessly integrated solutions for fitness, health care, and other areas with continuous research activities focused on surmounting obstacles and pursuing new opportunities [13].

6.2 Properties of MXene for Wearables

Emerging as a leader in wearable technology applications, MXene materials have a special set of characteristics that make them ideal for these kinds of applications [14]. Their exceptional conductivity guarantees effective signal transmission, which is essential for wearable devices that monitor environmental or health conditions [15]. One of MXenes' main advantages is their flexibility, which enables these materials to adapt to the changing shapes of the human body without sacrificing functionality. MXenes are incredibly robust despite their thinness; they can survive regular wear and tear. Their lightweight design and thin profile improve wearer comfort, which is important for gadgets that are intended to be worn all the time [16]. Furthermore, MXenes are biocompatible, which means that they won't harm human skin or implantable devices when utilized. MXenes' large surface area makes them highly sensitive and responsive, which is essential for the precise tracking and monitoring capabilities needed in wearable technology. All of these characteristics make MXenes a very promising material for the upcoming wearable technology. Below, some of these properties are discussed in detail.

6.2.1 Electrical Conductivity

Within the domain of wearable sensing, materials that may alter their electrical conductivity while responding to outside stimuli are very popular. For sensing materials to display this kind of activity, they must have a high electrical conductivity. Because most MXene combinations show semiconductor activity and the majority are projected to have metallic conductivity, the introduction of MXenes created several new opportunities in the field of wearable sensing technology [17]. The electrical properties of MXene are closely related to the surface functional groups. Higher work functions are produced by the high electronegativity of the fluorine and oxygen groups, whereas the substantial surface dipole moment of hydroxyl functionalization results in an ultra-low work function. Remarkably, on certain transition metals, a band can emerge simply by adjusting the surface functional groups. At the Fermi level, by offsetting the density states, electrical conductivity and band structure are among the functional groups that can be modified. For example, transition metals from d^1 (i.e., Y and Sc) show semiconducting behavior at any surface termination, but transition metals from d^2 (Hf, Zr, and Ti) need termination of oxygen for starting the bandgap. Additionally, MXene's electrical conductivity is influenced by the structural flaws and mixed surface groups that were introduced at the time of synthesis. Furthermore, intercalation of the Li^+ cations yield superior conductivity than organic intercalation, and so the method of intercalation and the process of etching could also affect MXene's conductivity. The electronic transport in MXene-based films may also be impacted by the flake size. The accurate accordance of two-dimensional sheets combined with MXene's high electrical conductivity makes the piezoresistive sensor system appropriate for wearable sensing technology [18].

6.2.2 Hydrophilicity

A key component of MXenes' usefulness and functionality, especially when it comes to wearable sensors, is their hydrophilicity. It speaks about a material's propensity to interact with or absorb water. This characteristic holds great importance for MXenes for multiple reasons, particularly when considering wearable sensors that frequently come into touch with human skin or are subjected to diverse biological fluids. The increased sensitivity of MXenes as sensors is partly attributed to their hydrophilic character. The capacity of MXene-based sensors to easily interact with biofluids, including water, guarantees that the sensors can detect even the smallest changes in the fluids' composition when employed for physiological parameter monitoring, such as sweat analysis. They are, therefore, very helpful for monitoring health indicators in real time [19].

It guarantees improved compatibility and interaction between biological elements—such as proteins and other biomolecules found in perspiration or on the surface of the skin—and MXene surfaces. For biosensors that use the identification of certain biomarkers for disease detection, health monitoring, or even environmental exposure to toxic compounds, this enhanced interface is essential. The hydrophilic surfaces of MXenes aid in the electron transport between the analyte and the sensor in electrochemical sensors. This is crucial for sensors that use redox reactions to detect chemical changes because water molecules can mediate and speed up these electron transfer processes, improving sensor response times and accuracy [20].

The way water molecules interact with the hydrophilic MXene layers can affect how flexible the material is and how well it conforms to various surfaces and shapes without losing its usefulness. Lastly, MXenes' processability, that is, how quickly they can be incorporated into or across a variety of substrates and matrices to create wearable sensors, is influenced by their hydrophilicity. Their preference for water can be used to advantage in processing methods such as hydrogel integration or solution processing, enabling the creation of a variety of wearable and efficient sensor systems [21].

6.2.3 Potential to Form Free-Standing Film

Investigating layered materials' two-dimensional (2D) characteristics requires separating them into separate sheets. Because MXene's interlayer bonds are stronger than those of materials like graphite or MoS_2, it can be stacked to create flexible films with exceptional electrochemical and piezoresistive properties. A colloidal solution of thin MXene layers can be formed during

MXene synthesis by using large organic bases or polar chemical molecules as intercalating agents. These can be filtered to create a homogeneous film that is perfect for wearable sensors since it offers great electrical conductivity and flexibility once it has dried. The unusual 2D structure of these MXene 'paper' films allows for the adjustment of their thickness and conductivity, offering a versatile platform for sensor design [22].

6.2.4 Mechanical Strength

Adhesive patches, elastomers, smart textiles, and other flexible and elastic substrates can all be combined with MXene-based pressure sensors. Because of their mechanical flexibility, the sensors can follow the natural curves of the body, making them pleasant and undetectable to wear while engaging in a variety of activities. Pressure sensors based on MXene have a broad dynamic range that makes it possible to record both high- and low-pressure levels. Because of their adaptability, they can be used to track a variety of activities, from minor posture adjustments to vigorous physical activity like running or jumping [23,24].

6.2.5 Fast Response Time and Long-Term Stability

Pressure sensors based on MXene have quick reaction times and provide immediate feedback on changes in pressure. Applications like gait analysis, sports performance tracking, and fall detection in the elderly that need quick detection of pressure differences depend on this quick response time. The superior mechanical stability and durability of MXene materials guarantee the long-term functionality of pressure sensors in wearable technology. For extended monitoring of pressure distribution during daily activities, rehabilitation exercises, or physical therapy sessions, this stability is necessary [25].

Wearable MXene-based pressure monitoring systems have a wide range of uses in sports, health care, and rehabilitation. These gadgets can be used for fall prevention, pressure ulcer prevention, gait analysis, posture monitoring, and athlete performance optimization. Furthermore, MXene-based pressure sensors can be incorporated into assistive technology for people with limited mobility, offering real-time feedback on pressure distribution, and averting accidents caused by pressure [26].

6.3 Fabrication Process of the MXene Sensing Layer

Sensor fabrication techniques for materials like MXenes involve a series of steps and methodologies aimed at creating devices that can detect physical, chemical, or biological changes. These techniques are crucial for integrating MXenes into wearable sensors, capitalizing on their unique properties such as high conductivity, flexibility, and strong electrochemical performance [27]. Below are some common sensor fabrication techniques, including those applicable to MXenes and other advanced materials.

6.3.1 Spin Coating

This is a method where a solution of the sensor material is deposited on a substrate and then spun at high speeds. This process evenly spreads the material across the substrate, forming thin films. It is particularly useful for creating uniform layers of MXenes for sensors.

6.3.2 Inkjet Printing

This technique involves ejecting small droplets of sensor material 'ink' onto a substrate in a controlled pattern. It allows for precise deposition of materials like MXene inks, making it suitable for flexible and wearable sensors where complex patterns or multilayer structures are needed [28].

6.3.3 Dip Coating

In this technique, the substrate is dipped into a liquid that contains the sensor material, and then withdrawn at a steady rate. As the solvent evaporates, a thin film is formed. Dip coating can be used for MXene materials to create layers with controlled thickness [29].

6.3.4 Layer-by-Layer Assembly

This is a technique for fabricating multilayer structures by alternately depositing positively and negatively charged layers of materials. For MXenes, which may have charged surfaces, this method can help in building up layered sensor components with enhanced sensitivity and selectivity.

Apart from this, electrospinning is also a process where a high-voltage charge is used to draw fine fibers from a liquid. This method can produce nanofiber mats of MXenes or composite materials, which are useful for developing sensors with porosity and a high surface area. Similarly, microcontact printing is a soft lithography technique where a stamp is employed for transferring the micropatterns of the sensor material onto substrates. While more common for materials like graphene, CVD can be adapted for certain types of MXenes. It involves depositing gaseous reactants onto a heated substrate, where they react or decompose to form a solid material. This method can produce high-quality, continuous films. Screen printing, stamping, blade coating, etc. are the methods of fabricating MXene layers [30]. Figure 6.1 briefly illustrates the different fabrication processes of MXene-based wearables

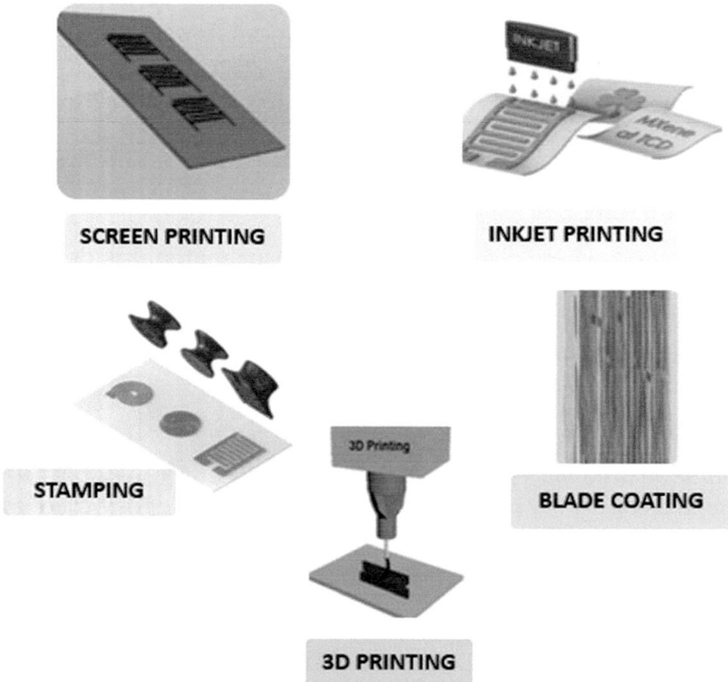

FIGURE 6.1
Different fabrication processes of MXene-based wearables.

6.4 Applications of MXene-Based Wearables

6.4.1 Physical Sensors

6.4.1.1 Pulse Monitoring

The most fundamental indicator of clinical life is the arterial pulse, which is felt via arterial palpation as a result of the aortic valve opening and shutting. An educated fingertip can detect the pulse of an artery in several parts of the body, such as the knee, groin, wrist, and neck. The heart rate is determined by measuring the arterial pulse per minute [31]. A pulse wave is made up of two main parts: (i) the diastolic component, which originates from the systolic component and (ii) relaxation of the heart, which is the wave that moves ahead when the heart contracts. The tidal waves that occur during systole, the dicrotic peak that arises during diastole, and percussion make up a typical pulse waveform [32]. These waves offer important details on the functions of the heart. Information about an individual's age, activity level, and heart-related conditions can be obtained by analysis of various pulse components. Nowadays, a variety of sensor types, including capacitive, infrared, piezoresistive, and piezoelectric sensors, are employed for capturing the signals of the pulse that operate on specific functional strategies. Arterial pulse detection was accomplished with excellent sensitivity and precision using MXene strain sensors based on the concept of piezoresistivity [33]. Several fabrication techniques were used for developing MXene-based pulse detectors. The MXene-based tattoo sensor's reaction with respect to the strain variations brought on the arterial pulse. The single-stranded MXene films were laser-patterned to create an ultrathin sensor that was extremely skin-conformal and sensitive to the arterial pulse. Zhang et al. used strain sensors based on polymer composites and MXene to show pulse detection. In this work, MXene was combined with crystal clay, a mixture of water, PVA, and dehydrating agents, to create a composite hydrogel [34]. The so-called M-hydrogel demonstrated outstanding stretchability, good adherence to human skin, and the capacity to heal itself. Good elastic characteristics and stretchability were achieved by the formation of a network of densely packed polymer chains within a clay matrix because of the presence of functional groups in the conductive filler MXene. Additionally, hydrogen bonding is promoted by the abundance of functional groups inside the structure of the composite, which aids in adhesion and self-healing qualities. The radial artery pulse was measured by mounting the M-hydrogel applied to the wrist. The pulse waves strained the hydrogel, modifying the electrical resistance of the MXene sheets by increasing or decreasing their contact area. In parallel, the ability of an MXene/RGO aerogel to sense the arterial pulse was investigated [35]. This aerogel was created as a piezoresistive strain sensor utilizing a freeze-drying technique. The ability to record a pulse and accurately differentiate between diastolic and percussion waves was made possible by this sensor's quick response time and excellent sensitivity. When the sensor was applied to the neck, it was likewise successful in tracking the jugular venous pulse. Shi et al. reported on another study involving an MXene-based pulse sensor, in which a bricks-and-mortar-fabricated sensor was utilized to capture the pulse of a human artery [36]. The screen printing was done by inks made up of Ti_3C_2-Ag NW-PDA/Ni^+ gel on a polyurethane substrate made up of the sensing element. The sensors demonstrated an inflated gauge factor for measuring pressure readings. This incredibly small and flexible sensor was precisely placed on the wrist, and it recorded the exact percussion, tidal, and diastolic components of a single heartbeat. MXene was used to construct wearable sensors that were both extremely sensitive and reproducible. However, it is crucial to combine single-use sensors with eco-friendly packaging materials for continual monitoring. According to reports, a biodegradable wearable sensor based on MXene can remain stable for a maximum of 2 weeks. Long-term use-oriented sensors were fabricated on sturdy substrates with durable packaging. Because of their great sensitivity and broad range of strain sensing, they can therefore use a single sensor for several different applications. Figure 6.2 illustrates artery pulse sensing using MXene.

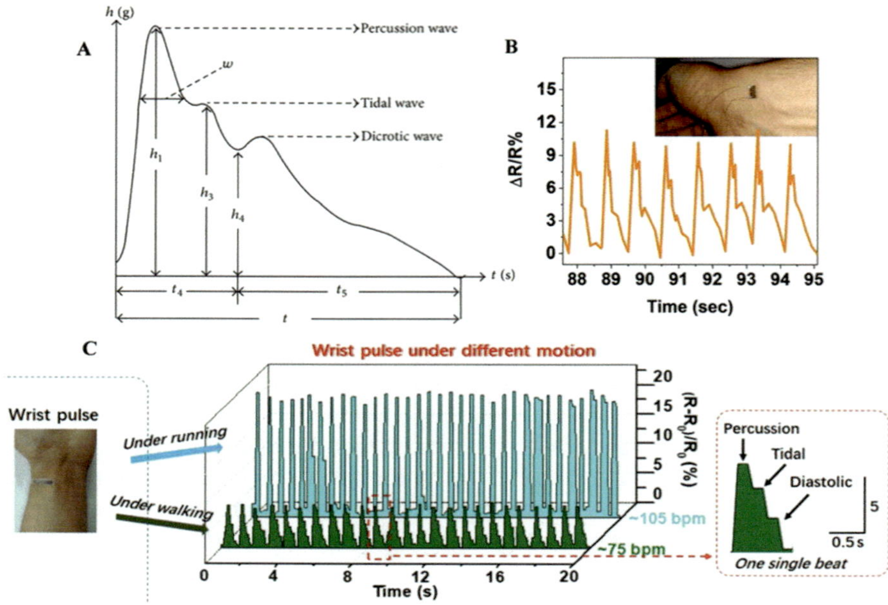

FIGURE 6.2
Artery pulse sensing using MXene [37].

6.4.1.2 Human Activity Monitoring

Human muscle movements and electrical activity are tracked by electromyography (EMG), which is crucial for several biomedical applications. Additionally, it is essential for sports and prosthetic applications, which may open doors for human–machine interfaces in robotics [38]. Furthermore, body-mounted strain sensors provide precise monitoring of different muscle actions. Because carbon nanotubes (CNTs) and graphene have remarkable electrical and physical properties, their discovery has completely changed the field of flexible and wearable sensing [39]. These materials' excellent electrical conductivity and pliability made it easier to construct intricate devices on flexible substrates. Multiple conducting channels are created for the passage of electrons by the highly linked network structure formed by the 1D CNTs. The network structure flexes when strain is applied, adjusting the sensing layer's resistance by the strain that is created. In addition, this technique offers higher sensitivity than thin-film metal strain gauges. Accordingly, the sensitivity and working range of the sensor are affected by the orientation of the CNTs. Flexible strain sensors based on graphene were created using a similar method. When under tension, graphene's conductive two-dimensional layers move over one another. The conducting pathways were altered by the shift in the overlapping region, which changed the sensor resistance [40]. The capacity to sense strain effectively at higher values was increased by flexible graphene monolayers because they gave the sensor layer superior mechanical strength. By creating graphene–CNT composite sensors, the benefits of CNTs and graphene were coupled to provide increased sensitivity, a broad operating range, and a robust construction. Similarly, MXene's strong electrical conductivity helps create sensors with greater flexibility by using it as a filler in polymer composites [41]. The technology that allows the MXene sensor to react to strain is piezoresistivity. Strain is applied to a sensor when it is moved relative to a particular area of the body. The flexible MXene layer is mechanically deformed by this strain, which modifies the electron conduction paths. The applied strain directly correlates with the change in the sensor's electrical resistance. Numerous metrics are used in human activity monitoring, including voice recognition, gesture recognition, facial expression detection, arm and leg movements, and foot tracking. While the movements of joints and muscles of the legs and hands necessitate the recording of elevated strain values, facial expression and vocal cord motions are classified as lower strain regimens. Figure 6.3 explains the possible human monitoring activities of MXene. To assess a variety of bodily movements, sensors must have a broad sensing range and good sensitivity at low strain values. Below is a discussion of a couple of these applications.

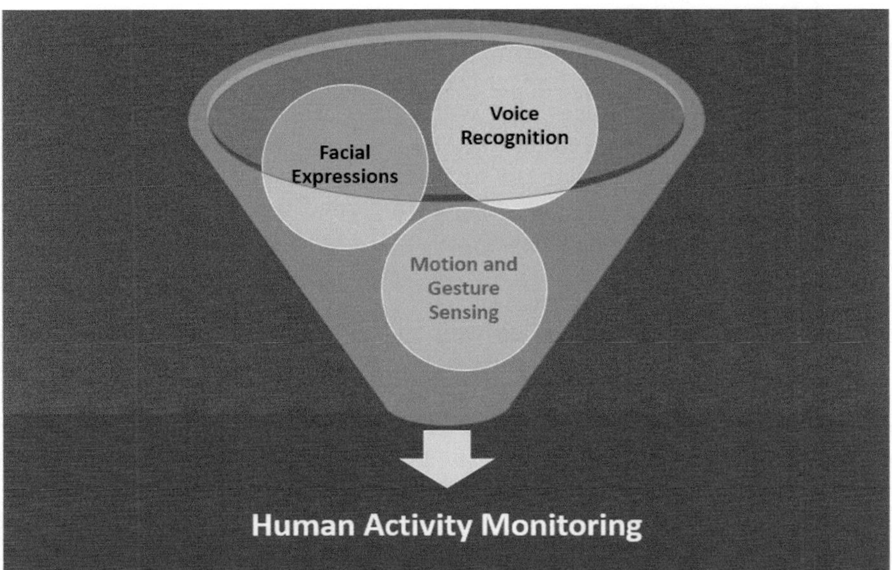

FIGURE 6.3
Possible human monitoring activities of MXene.

(i) Facial Expressions

Facial expressions are the movements of muscles beneath the skin of the face, mostly used to portray emotions. Different facial expressions are created by combining several facial muscles. It would be advantageous for developing technology in the areas of robotics, human–machine interfaces, and machine learning to comprehend and research these expressions. Furthermore, biomedical uses for tracking an individual's expression include tracking the recuperation from neurological injuries, paralysis, etc. The expression of emotions in this situation is greatly aided by eye movement. A sensor made up of MXene-based material was affixed to the edge of the eye to monitor eyelid closing and opening. This allowed for the analysis of the blinking rate to ascertain the veracity of a statement. Furthermore, the major emotional states of human happiness and sadness were studied through the motions of the cheeks using an MXene strain sensor. There was also mention of a pressure sensor that was placed on the cheek to track occlusion [42].

(ii) Voice Recognition

Vocal cords are used by humans to make sounds to communicate and convey emotions. Air is pumped from the vocal cords and vibrates, and the lungs, and articulators like the lips, cheek, and tongue, modulate and direct the voice according to the situation in which it is produced. Sound is a necessary byproduct of speaking, singing, yelling, screaming, and other activities. To decode and interpret the information that humans emit in various frequencies, microphones are typically utilized to record, transform, and understand those frequencies. It is noteworthy to consider that the strain sensors on the neck may identify voice patterns; MXene sensors are then affixed to the neck to investigate various noises. The wearable sensor experiences strain from the movement of the vocal cords and Adam's apple, which changes the resistance and creates distinct patterns for various words. For medical purposes, the act of swallowing and gulping was recorded using the MXene sensor. Breathing variations were also detected by the neck-mounted sensor [29].

(iii) Motion and Gesture Sensing

In human–machine interfaces as well as medical and sports applications that track muscle damage recovery, fractures, and other conditions, gesture sensing plays a critical role. Muscles and joints move often and in a variety of ways during motion detection. Such applications require a flexible and extremely durable sensor. The sensor package should be able to suppress noise from a variety of other factors, including temperature and perspiration. With the help of the exceptional properties of nanomaterials like graphene and carbon nanotubes, a broad range of motion sensors have been created. Because of their potential uses in stretchy electronics, flexible and wearable smart fabrics are becoming increasingly common in the motion tracking and healthcare industries. Kedambaimoole et al.'s recent work showed how to fabricate flexible sensors out of graphene for use in gesture detection applications. Human motion detection was investigated using a very stretchy sensor made of dry-spun carbon nanotubes on an Ecoflex substrate [43,44].

Researchers now have new methods to construct pressure and strain sensors because of the development of MXene. Motion and gesture sensing were studied with these sensors. A 3D hybrid sponge covered with MXene was employed as a strain sensor for detecting the movements of fingers. The joints of the fingers were attached to the sensor, and as the fingers bent, the current was recorded. They also illustrate how a sensor developed by the composites of MXene–hydrogels affixed to the fingertips and joints was able to recognize motions. Due to the great sensitivity, versatility, and broad variety of strain-measuring potential of MXene-based sensors, a thorough assessment of behavior among individuals might be extensively investigated. Such sensors can forecast a patient's future state of health. For example, an MXene-based pressure sensor is affixed to the muscles of the arm to identify contractions of the radial muscle that result from fist motions. They work to aid healing muscle injury and physical training. Furthermore, it has been claimed that flexible MXene sensors sealed with transparent tape and affixed to elbow joints and muscles (functions of orthopedics) may easily record the bending–straightening of joints. Additionally, because of its reliability, which shows the I vs. T in reaction to ankle-bending, produced reliable evaluations. Large strain changes occur when knee bending is monitored while walking to assess posture, and these types of sensors require an elevated stretchability and functioning range. When jogging or performing other more strenuous activities, the $Ti_3C_2T_x$-Ag NW-PDA/N^{2+} composite-based sensors made using a design of mortar-and-motor accurately calculate the signals of motion [36]. The sensor was used to track the steps taken by a woman walking at a pace of 40 steps/min and jogging at 80 steps/min. The sensor was installed on the knee. Addressing numerous overlooked issues may be made possible by concentrating on the particular application for in-depth research and making use of the know-how technique of MXene-based sensors. Therefore, adding motion-sensing devices to the body that can gather and interpret a wide range of biomonitoring data is an appealing option.

6.4.2 Chemical Sensors

6.4.2.1 Electrochemical Sensors

The non-intrusive assessment of electrolytes or metabolites using human bodily fluids, such as saliva, sweat, etc., is gaining popularity. Electrochemical wearable sensors offer the ability to continually assess biochemical markers of persons that aid in maintaining health and fitness, such as electrolytes, cortisol, pH, glucose, etc., in comparison to physical sensors. Wearable applications can safely utilize electrochemical sensors because of their low potential operation and consequently low power consumption. They are also good candidates for body mounting due to their simplicity in downsizing, affordability, quick response time, and adaptability in interfacing with wearable electronics. Transducer materials are crucial for achieving certain sensor functioning goals, such as detection limit, selectivity, sensitivity, etc., for creating wearable electrochemical devices. In this section, we cover the electrochemical characteristics of $Ti_3C_2T_x$ MXene [45]. Wearable electrochemical sensor design and fabrication require an understanding of these features as well as the sensing mechanism. Electrodes are essentially used by electrochemical sensors to convert the reaction from chemical to electrical output. Transducer materials are also utilized for enhancing the functionality of such electrodes and effectively immobilize bioreceptors (enzymes, antibodies, aptamers, etc.) without interfering with their activity. Consequently, it is anticipated that transducer materials will have a high electrical conductivity to detect minute electrical fluctuations at the electrode–electrolyte interface [46].

As far as we know, only one research work has used electrochemical technology based on $Ti_3C_2T_x$ MXene for wearable sensor applications. Within this study, incredibly effective electrochemical indicators to detect lactate and glucose in sweat were Prussian blue composites and $Ti_3C_2T_x$ MXene. Because sweat lacks oxygen, one of the main problems with enzyme sensors based on perspiration is their low sensibility and narrow detecting region. To overcome these problems, a biosensing patch (electrode) based on the solid–liquid–air interface was created utilizing the CNTs/Ti_3C_2/PB electrode (the CNTs serve as mechanical support). Carbon fiber membrane (CFM) was used to support the patch, which helped to allow the oxygen to permeate from the biosensor patch's bottom to its top while preventing the electrode from getting wet, which is where the enzymes were rendered inert. The enzymes mounted over electrodes (CNTs/$Ti_3C_2T_x$/PB/CFMs) were provided with a continual oxygen-rich environment through the formation of a solid–liquid–air interface through the reaction with the solution of the analyte. Superior stability and sensitivity (11.4 mA $mm^{-1}cm^{-2}$ for lactate and 35.3 mA mm^{-1} cm^{-2} for glucose) were the outcomes.

(i) Sweat Analysis

Sweat analysis is an effective method to provide details on a person's physical condition. In addition to water, sweat also contains important indicators such as protein, potassium, calcium, chlorine, sodium, urea, lactate, glucose, etc. These biomarkers can be examined to learn more about an individual's health, which is crucial for both sports and medical diagnosis. Perspiration is secreted by sweat glands beneath the skin. As a result, sweat sensors are typically applied topically as tattoos or patches. For the sensor to produce good skin adherence, it must be skin-conformal and biocompatible. Sweat sensors have several issues, including limited sensitivity, extended response

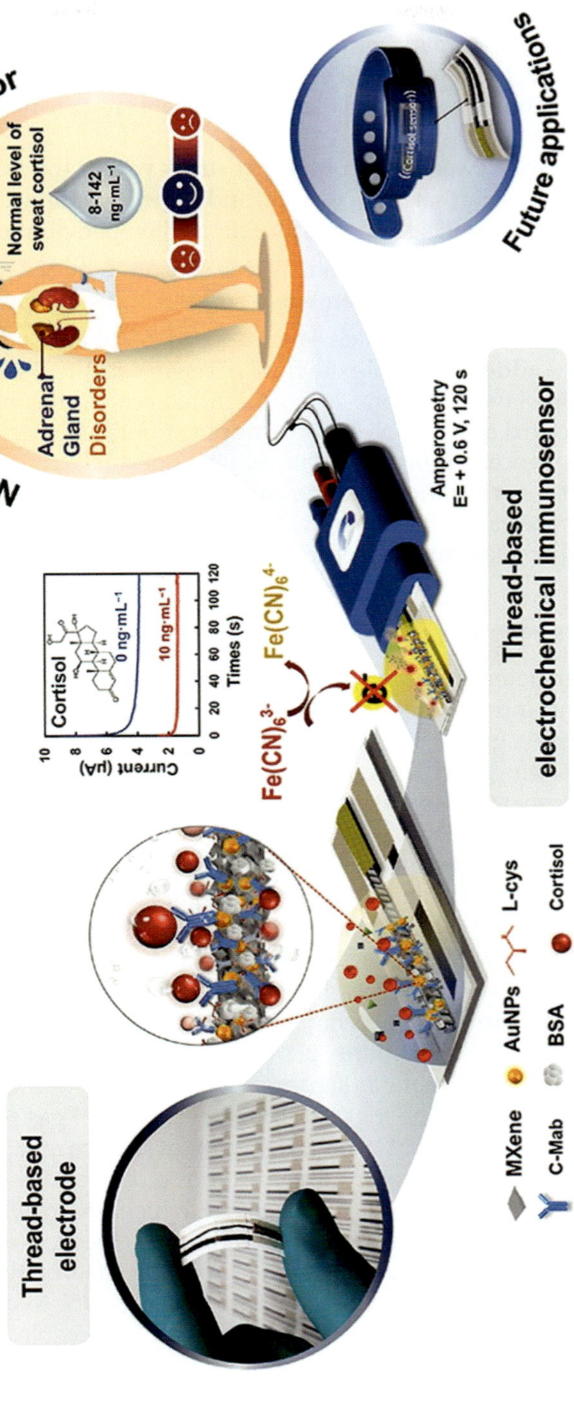

FIGURE 6.4
Schematic view of sweat analysis with the help of an electrochemical immunosensor [47].

times, decreased shelf lives, degradation with frequent use, and simultaneous assessment of many biomarkers. For the first time, Lei et al. [46] used MXene to develop a wearable sweat sensor that could measure pH, glucose, and lactate. The three-layered electrochemical sensor is made up of:

(i) A layer of sweat absorption that sticks within the skin and is made of porous fabric that collects sweat and serpentine tunnels. Sensors measure the levels of pH, glucose, and lactate when perspiration builds up.
(ii) Sensing layer: this is where active sensors with sensor gaps and spiral tunnels carved into them are inserted.
(iii) The cover layer, which is composed of pliable silicon rubber with pores added to enable the flow of oxygen in the direction of the active sensor layer. The one in question aids in protecting the outside air. In regard to wearable sensing applications, MXenes' exceptional solution processability, 2D nature, and conductivity open the door for their incorporation into the current electrochemical system. Figure 6.4 provides a schematic view of sweat analysis with the help of an electrochemical immunosensor.

6.4.2.2 Gas Sensors

The regular deterioration according to the index of the air quality in emerging nations and large cities makes wearable gas monitors imperative. Toxic and dangerous gases must be detected in a variety of industrial and environmental settings, which requires constant and real-time gas monitoring. Although research into gas sensors has been ongoing for some time, wearability is a relatively new feature that offers various benefits for applications including risk assessment and health monitoring. Wearability can be attained by the creation of adaptable, biocompatible sensors that maintain the detecting features [48]. High sensitivity, quick reaction time, a broad range of detection across various concentrations and gases, strong gas-specific selectivity, and capacity to identify the molecules of gas and chemical vapors at very low rates are the main characteristics of gas sensors. Due to the extraordinary features they inherit, 2D materials have attracted a great deal of interest in the creation of gas sensors. Currently, one of the 2D materials that has been investigated the most for the applications of gas sensing is MXenes. The layered structure of MXenes offers a lot of surface area for the adsorption of gas molecules. An increased signal-to-noise ratio and better sensitivity are facilitated by good metal-like conductivity, which occurs when gas molecules adsorb physically and chemically, changing the electrical response. They are very appealing candidates for gas sensing because of the strong binding that the numerous surface functional groups produce to analyte molecules. MXene is perfect for gas detection because of its flexible surface chemistry and many sites of adsorption. This material's hydrophilicity and flexibility facilitate wearable application adaption. Although a number of MXenes are investigated for gas sensing, this chapter especially addresses the application of $Ti_3C_2T_x$ [49].

The two major methods of sensing that have been seen in MXene-based gas sensors are modification of the Schottky barrier (SB) and the adsorbed gas molecules' surface charge transfer. The electrical resistance of the sensing film changes as a result of gas molecules adhering to the active defect sites and surfaces of functionalized Ti_3C_2. The majority of charge carriers of film and the analytes' electron-donating/withdrawing characteristics are what cause this shift in resistance. The presence of the Schottky barrier (SB) could notably increase the sensitivity of gas. For instance, powerful oxidizing gases could push the SB upward and obstruct the flow of electrons in a sensor material where electrons serve as mobility carriers, thus enhancing the sensitivity to gas.

According to Lee et al., wearable gas sensors based on Ti_3C_2 were created and placed on a flexible polyimide substrate to detect volatile organic compounds (VOCs) [50]. At room temperature, the chemiresistive sensor demonstrated great sensitivity when exposed to a variety of polar gases, including methanol, ammonia gas, acetone, and ethanol. The Ti_3C_2 sensor exhibited p-type sensing activity, responding more strongly to acetone gas and ammonia gas, respectively. MXene/graphene hybrid fibers were created by Lee for NH_3 sensing. A scalable wet spinning technique was used to develop flexible and stable MXene/rGO fibers. These fibers were woven on laboratory aprons for the demonstration of their exceptional resilience against mechanical deformations and potential for gas-sensing applications in wearables. Compared to the conventional rigid films, the moldable/flexible fibers are shaped within a large surface-to-volume ratio which demonstrates a three-order better sensitivity toward gas sensing. A Ti_3C_2 MXene-CPAM nanocomposite (cationic polyacrylamide) for flexible NH_3 gas sensors was described by Zhao et al. in a related study [51]. These sensors showed great adaptability for wearable applications, long-term stability at ambient temperature, and remarkable selectivity toward ammonia. In addition to improving the mechanical stability of a sort of weak Ti_3C_2 MXene, the inclusion of CPAM also significantly boosted the composite material's overall NH_3 sensitivity due to the numerous surface functional groups of CPAM and the formation of hydrogen bonds with the analyte gas. The compatibility of MXene and composite materials for wearable applications can be additionally researched, as multiple researchers have reported on their capacity to sense a range of gases.

6.5 Future Prospects

Because of their hydrophilic properties and robust water-based ink production, MXenes are a novel class of 2D materials that exhibit promise in wearables. Their surfactant-free colloidal solutions increase their adaptability in device creation, including different printing methods. Their tunable rheological characteristics allow for the fabrication of sensors using additive manufacturing, and their capacity to create free-standing films provides flexible design options. Because of its metallic conductivity and hydrophilicity, Ti_3C_2-MXene is a great filler for polymeric composites. The piezoresistive feature of MXene is used to create strain sensors with excellent sensitivity, a broad operating range, and quick response times for wearable applications. MXene sensors show promise for real-time healthcare monitoring and human motion detection when paired with wireless transmitters. Furthermore, highly sensitive humidity detection could be provided by multifunctional textiles using MXene sensors while preserving flexibility and porosity. MXenes have the potential to be used in military applications as an electromagnetic interference barrier.

When compared to graphene-based sensors, MXene's wearable applications are still in their infancy, despite encouraging research. The manufacturing of flexible MXene-based devices has not received much attention. By using polymer composites with different biocompatible polymers to address the stretchability issue, MXene's uses may be expanded. Industrial-scale use of fabrication techniques like 3D printing and extrusion printing could hasten the development of wearable sensors. MXene has the potential to be used in gas sensing for environmental monitoring because it has low detection limits and great sensitivity to volatile organic chemicals. Hybrid MXene-gas sensors may improve the performance of wearable sensors. All things considered, MXene sensors have a wide range of possible uses if their properties are tuned. However, to fully utilize MXene's potential in wearable technology, more investigation and development are required.

MXenes provide a flexible framework for the functionalization and immobilization of bioreceptors, enabling the development of sensors that can identify a range of analytes, including cancer biomarkers, glucose, lactate, and hemoglobin. MXenes are unique among 2D nanomaterials because of their strong conductivity, electrochemical activity, photothermal sensitivity, biocompatibility, and flexibility. These characteristics make it possible to create wearable sensors that can measure physiological and physical factors directly from perspiration. Although $Ti_3C_2T_x$ MXenes have been used as transducer materials for biomarker detection, the majority of sensors that have been described up to this point are not able to be attached to the body, suggesting unrealized potential for the creation of extremely sensitive wearable electrochemical sensors. Recent developments include the use of MXene in the elimination of urea, which makes it easier to detect urea in sweat without the need for an enzyme. This could help discover disorders connected to the kidneys early on and monitor the health of important organs. Moreover, MXenes' catalytic and self-reducing qualities present chances for integration with metals and polymers to improve sensor performance, thereby streamlining the manufacturing process for wearable electrochemical sensors that can run on their own. MXene electrochemical sensors could be useful to athletes in detecting doping and tracking stress levels.

6.6 Conclusion

In conclusion, MXene-based materials hold tremendous potential for revolutionizing the landscape of wearable device applications. Throughout this chapter, we have explored the diverse range of functionalities and properties that make MXenes highly attractive for wearable technology. From their exceptional electrical conductivity and mechanical flexibility to their biocompatibility and chemical stability, MXenes offer a compelling combination of characteristics that address key requirements for wearable device applications.

Despite the significant promise of MXenes, several challenges remain to be addressed, including scalability of synthesis, integration with flexible substrates, and ensuring long-term stability and biocompatibility. However, these challenges also present opportunities for further research and innovation in the field. By tackling these obstacles and exploring new avenues for advancement, MXene-based materials can fulfill their potential as enabling technologies for wearable devices.

Looking ahead, interdisciplinary collaborations between materials scientists, engineers, and biomedical researchers will be essential for driving progress in MXene-based wearable device applications. By leveraging the unique properties of MXenes and developing innovative solutions, we can envision a future where wearable devices seamlessly integrate into our daily lives, offering personalized, connected, and transformative experiences for health care, fitness monitoring, communication, and beyond. MXene-based materials represent a promising frontier in wearable technology, poised to shape the future of human–computer interaction and personalized health care. With continued research and development efforts, MXenes have the potential to unlock new possibilities and applications, enriching our lives and enhancing the way we interact with the world around us.

References

1. A. J. Bandodkar and J. Wang, Non-invasive wearable electrochemical sensors: A review, *Trends in Biotechnology*, 2014, 32(7), 363–371
2. S. C. Mukhopadhyay, Wearable sensors for human activity monitoring: A review, *IEEE Sensors Journal*, 2014, 15(3), 1321–1330.

3. J. T. Reeder, Y. Xue, D. Franklin, Y. Deng, J. Choi, O. Prado, R. Kim, C. Liu, J. Hanson and J. Ciraldo, Resettable skin interfaced microfluidic sweat collection devices with chemesthetic hydration feedback, *Nature Communications*, 2019, 10(1), 1–12.
4. V. Shirhatti, S. Nuthalapati, V. Kedambaimoole, S. Kumar, M. M. Nayak and K. Rajanna, Laser-patterned multifunctional sensor array with graphene nanosheets as a smart biomonitoring fashion accessory. arXiv preprint, 2021, arXiv:2104.01615.
5. J. C. Yang, J. Mun, S. Y. Kwon, S. Park, Z. Bao and S. Park, Electronic skin: Recent progress and future prospects for skin-attachable devices for health monitoring, robotics, and prosthetics, *Advanced Materials*, 2019, 31(48), 1904765.
6. X. Wang, L. Dong, H. Zhang, R. Yu, C. Pan and Z. L. Wang, Recent progress in electronic skin, *Advanced Science*, 2015, 2(10), 1500169.
7. D.-H. Kim, N. Lu, R. Ma, Y.-S. Kim, R.-H. Kim, S. Wang, J. Wu, S. M. Won, H. Tao and A. Islam, Epidermal electronics, *Science*, 2011, 333(6044), 838–843.
8. Z. Ma, D. Kong, L. Pan and Z. Bao, Skin-inspired electronics: Emerging semiconductor devices and systems, *Journal of Semiconductors*, 2020, 41(4), 041601.
9. S. Kabiri Ameri, R. Ho, H. Jang, L. Tao, Y. Wang, L. Wang, D. M. Schnyer, D. Akinwande and N. Lu, Graphene electronic tattoo sensors, *American Chemical Society Nano*, 2017, 11(8), 7634–7641.
10. C. Choi, Y. Lee, K. W. Cho, J. H. Koo and D.-H. Kim, Wearable and implantable soft bioelectronics using two-dimensional materials, *Accounts of Chemical Research*, 2018, 52(1), 73–81.
11. B. Anasori, M. R. Lukatskaya and Y. Gogotsi, 2D metal carbides and nitrides (MXenes) for energy storage, *Nature Reviews Materials*, 2017, 2(2), 1–17.
12. K. Chaturvedi, V. Hada, S. Paul, B. Sarma, D. Malvi, M. Dhangar, H. Bajpai, A. Singhwane, A. K. Srivastava and S. Verma, The rise of MXene: A wonder 2D material, from its synthesis and properties to its versatile applications—A comprehensive review, *Topics in Current Chemistry*, 2023, 381(2), 11.
13. Singhwane A, Chaturvedi K, Mohapatra RK, Srivastava AK, Verma S. Mxene-based composite materials as antibacterial agents for healthcare applications. In Age of MXenes, Volume 2. Applications in Diagnostics, Therapeutics, and Environmental Remediation 2023. American Chemical Society, 2023, pp. 1–17.
14. C. Ma, M. G. Ma, C. Si, X. X. Ji and P. Wan, Flexible Mxene-based composites for wearable devices, *Advanced Functional Materials*, 2021, 31(22), 2009524.
15. M. M. Hasan, M. M. Hossain and H. K. Chowdhury, Two-dimensional MXene-based flexible nanostructures for functional nanodevices: A review, *Journal of Materials Chemistry*, 2021, 9(6), 3231–3269.
16. N. Li, J. Peng, W.-J. Ong, T. Ma, P. Zhang, J. Jiang, X. Yuan and C. J. Zhang, MXenes: An emerging platform for wearable electronics and looking beyond, *Matter*, 2021, 4(2), 377–407.
17. H. Kim and H. N. Alshareef, MXetronics: MXene-enabled electronic and photonic devices, *ACS Materials Letters*, 2019, 2(1), 55–70.
18. M. Ghidiu, M. R. Lukatskaya, M.-Q. Zhao, Y. Gogotsi and M. W. Barsoum, Conductive two-dimensional titanium carbide 'clay' with high volumetric capacitance, *Nature*, 2014, 516(7529), 78–81.

19. H. Chen, Y. Wen, Y. Qi, Q. Zhao, L. Qu and C. Li, Pristine titanium carbide MXene films with environmentally stable conductivity and superior mechanical strength, *Advanced Functional Materials*, 2020, 30(5), 1906996.
20. S. Hajian, P. Khakbaz, M. Moshayedi, D. Maddipatla, B. B. Narakathu, V. S. Turkani, B. J. Bazuin, M. Pourfath and M. Z. Atashbar in Impact of Different Ratios of Fluorine, Oxygen, and Hydroxyl Surface Terminations on Ti_3C_2Tx MXene as Ammonia Sensor: A First-Principles Study, *IEEE SENSORS*, IEEE, 2018, pp. 1–4.
21. Y. Z. Zhang, Y. Wang, Q. Jiang, J. K. El-Demellawi, H. Kim and H. N. Alshareef, MXene printing and patterned coating for device applications, *Advanced Materials*, 2020, 32(21), 1908486.
22. T. Hu, M. Hu, Z. Li, H. Zhang, C. Zhang, J. Wang and X. Wang, Interlayer coupling in two-dimensional titanium carbide MXenes, *Physical Chemistry Chemical Physics*, 2016, 18(30), 20256–20260.
23. V. N. Borysiuk, V. N. Mochalin and Y. Gogotsi, Bending rigidity of two-dimensional titanium carbide (MXene) nanoribbons: A molecular dynamics study, *Computational Materials Science*, 2018, 143, 418–424.
24. A. Lipatov, H. Lu, M. Alhabeb, B. Anasori, A. Gruverman, Y. Gogotsi and A. Sinitskii, Elastic properties of 2D $Ti_3C_2T_x$ MXene monolayers and bilayers, *Science Advances*, 2018, 4(6), eaat0491.
25. X. Zhan, C. Si, J. Zhou and Z. Sun, MXene and MXene-based composites: Synthesis, properties and environment-related applications, *Nanoscale Horizons.*, 2020, 5, 235–258.
26. B. Anasori, M. R. Lukatskaya and Y. Gogotsi, 2D metal carbides and nitrides (MXenes) for energy storage, *Nature Reviews Materials*, 2017, 2, 16098.
27. B. Akuzum, K. Maleski, B. Anasori, P. Lelyukh, N. J. Alvarez, E. C. Kumbur and Y. Gogotsi, Rheological characteristics of 2D titanium carbide (MXene) dispersions: A guide for processing MXenes, *American Chemical Society Nano*, 2018, 12(3), 2685–2694.
28. M. Singh, H. M. Haverinen, P. Dhagat and G. E. Jabbour, Inkjet printing—process and its applications, *Advanced Materials*, 2010, 22(6), 673–685.
29. Y. Yue, N. Liu, W. Liu, M. Li, Y. Ma, C. Luo, S. Wang and J. Rao, 3D hybrid porous Mxene-sponge network and its application in piezoresistive sensor, *Nano Energy*, 2018, 50, 79–87.
30. Z. Chen, Z. Li, J. Li, C. Liu, C. Lao, Y. Fu, C. Liu, Y. Li, P. Wang and Y. He, 3D printing of ceramics: A review, *Journal of the European Ceramic Society*, 2019, 39(4), 661–687.
31. T. Yang, X. Jiang, Y. Zhong, X. Zhao, S. Lin, J. Li, X. Li, J. Xu, Z. Li and H. Zhu, A wearable and highly sensitive graphene strain sensor for precise home-based pulse wave monitoring, *ACS Sensors*, 2017, 2(7), 967–974.
32. H. Xu, J. Liu, J. Zhang, G. Zhou, N. Luo and N. Zhao, Flexible organic/inorganic hybrid near-infrared photoplethysmogram sensor for cardiovascular monitoring, *Advanced Materials*, 2017, 29(31), 1700975.
33. A. R. Maria, S. Pasca and R. Strungaru in *Heart Rate Monitoring by Using Non-invasive Wearable Sensor, E-Health and Bioengineering Conference (EHB)*, IEEE, 2017, pp. 587–590.
34. Y.-Z. Zhang, K. H. Lee, D. H. Anjum, R. Sougrat, Q. Jiang, H. Kim and H. N. Alshareef, MXenes stretch hydrogel sensor performance to new limits, *Science Advances*, 2018, 4(6), eaat0098.

35. Y. Ma, Y. Yue, H. Zhang, F. Cheng, W. Zhao, J. Rao, S. Luo, J. Wang, X. Jiang and Z. Liu, 3D synergistical MXene/ reduced graphene oxide aerogel for a piezoresistive sensor, *American Chemical Society Nano*, 2018, 12(4), 3209–3216.
36. X. Shi, H. Wang, X. Xie, Q. Xue, J. Zhang, S. Kang, C. Wang, J. Liang and Y. Chen, Bioinspired ultrasensitive and stretchable MXene-based strain sensor via nacre-mimetic microscale "brick-and-mortar" architecture, *American Chemical Society Nano*, 2018, 13(1), 649–659.
37. V. Kedambaimoole, K. Harsh, K. Rajanna, P. Sen, M. M. Nayak and S. Kumar, MXene wearables: Properties, fabrication strategies, sensing mechanism and applications, *Materials Advances*, 2022, 3(9), 3784–808.
38. T. Yamada, Y. Hayamizu, Y. Yamamoto, Y. Yomogida, Izadi-Najafabadi, D. N. Futaba and K. Hata, A stretchable carbon nanotube strain sensor for human-motion detection, *Nature Nanotechnology*, 2011, 6(5), 296.
39. J. Ren, C. Wang, X. Zhang, T. Carey, K. Chen, Y. Yin and F. Torrisi, Environmentally-friendly conductive cotton fabric as flexible strain sensor based on hot press reduced graphene oxide, *Carbon*, 2017, 111, 622–630.
40. J. Shi, X. Li, H. Cheng, Z. Liu, L. Zhao, T. Yang, Z. Dai, Z. Cheng, E. Shi and L. Yang, Graphene reinforced carbon nanotube networks for wearable strain sensors, *Advanced Functional Materials*, 2016, 26(13), 2078–2084.
41. J. Shi, J. Hu, Z. Dai, W. Zhao, P. Liu, L. Zhao, Y. Guo, T. Yang, L. Zou and K. Jiang, Graphene welded carbon nanotube crossbars for biaxial strain sensors, *Carbon*, 2017, 123, 786–793.
42. Y. Ma, N. Liu, L. Li, X. Hu, Z. Zou, J. Wang, S. Luo and Y. Gao, A highly flexible and sensitive piezoresistive sensor based on MXene with greatly changed interlayer distances, *Nature Communications*, 2017, 8(1), 1207.
43. S. Lim, D. Son, J. Kim, Y. B. Lee, J. K. Song, S. Choi, D. J. Lee, J. H. Kim, M. Lee and T. Hyeon, Transparent and stretchable interactive human machine interface based on patterned graphene heterostructures, *Advanced Functional Materials*, 2015, 25(3), 375–383.
44. M. Liu, X. Pu, C. Jiang, T. Liu, X. Huang, L. Chen, C. Du, J. Sun, W. Hu and Z. L. Wang, Large-area all-textile pressure sensors for monitoring human motion and physiological signals, *Advanced Materials*, 2017, 29(41), 1703700.
45. S. Verma, U. Dwivedi, K. Chaturvedi, N. Kumari, M. Dhangar, S. A. Hashmi, R. Singhal and A. K. Srivastava, Progress of 2D MXenes based composites for efficient electromagnetic interference shielding applications: A review, *Synthetic Metals*, 2022, 287, 117095.
46. Y. Lei, W. Zhao, Y. Zhang, Q. Jiang, J. H. He, J. Baeumner, O. S. Wolfbeis, Z. L. Wang, K. N. Salama and H. N. Alshareef, A MXene-based wearable biosensor system for high-performance in vitro perspiration analysis, *Small*, 2019, 15(19), 1901190.
47. T. Laochai, J. Yukird, N. Promphet, J. Qin, O. Chailapakul and N. Rodthongkum, Non-invasive electrochemical immunosensor for sweat cortisol based on L-cys/AuNPs/MXene modified thread electrode, *Biosensors and Bioelectronics*, 2022, 203, 114039.
48. A. Kaushik, R. Kumar, S. K. Arya, M. Nair, B. Malhotra and S. Bhansali, Organic–inorganic hybrid nanocomposite- based gas sensors for environmental monitoring, *Chemical Reviews*, 2015, 115(11), 4571–4606.

49. E. Lee, A. VahidMohammadi, B. C. Prorok, Y. S. Yoon, M. Beidaghi and D.-J. Kim, Room temperature gas sensing of two-dimensional titanium carbide (MXene), *ACS Applied Materials & Interfaces*, 2017, 9(42), 37184–37190.
50. S. H. Lee, W. Eom, H. Shin, R. B. Ambade, J. H. Bang, H. W. Kim and T. H. Han, Room-temperature, highly durable $Ti_3C_2T_x$ MXene/graphene hybrid fibers for NH3 gas sensing, *ACS Applied Materials & Interfaces*, 2020, 12(9), 10434–10442.
51. L. Zhao, Y. Zheng, K. Wang, C. Lv, W. Wei, L. Wang and W. Han, Highly stable cross-linked cationic polyacrylamide/$Ti_3C_2T_x$ MXene nanocomposites for flexible ammonia-recognition devices, *Advanced Materials Technologies*, 2020, 5(7), 2000248.

7

Emerging 2D Titanium Carbide MXene in Tissue Regeneration for Healthcare Applications

Anju Singhwane, Manal Khan, Ranjan Mohapatra,
Avanish Kumar Sriastava, and Sarika Verma

7.1 Introduction

On account of the exceptional electrical, mechanical, and visual properties of other 2D layered materials, their study has significantly increased since graphene's exfoliation [1,2]. Beyond graphene, the most extensively studied 2D materials include transition metal dichalcogenides, phosphorene, and its variants. The scientific community has recently paid intense attention to the determination of the 'MXenes' family of 2D layered compounds due to their unusual structural and electrical properties, enabling their usage in various possible applications [3]. In 2011, a MAX phase was chemically etched to reveal a novel class of materials called MXenes. This is a two-dimensional flake with the formula $M_n+1X_nT_x$ (n=1, 2, 3) that was left behind after the AA layer of a MAX phase was discarded. Surface termination, also known as TT, is most typically represented by (F), (OH), or (O) atoms. Because of their surface atom terminations, MXenes are a family of two-dimensional crystalline materials with a potentially uncountable range of diameter but thin breadth atomically. These materials differ from one another in terms of their features. Titanium carbide (Ti_3C_2) was the first MXene to be discovered. Since then, the topic has expanded as researchers have tried to understand the characteristics and uses of MXenes through studies. They are useful for biological applications, electromagnetic shielding, environmental applications like potable water, and energy storage. MXenes offer a possible alternative to the materials we now use. Among the many applications, the tissue regeneration property is a crucial area to focus on. The 2D titanium carbide MXene has the potential to aid in cell regeneration [4]. Additionally, it demonstrates remarkable and distinctive qualities, such as metal-like conductivity for heat

DOI: 10.1201/9781003353287-7

and electricity and ceramic qualities, including elastic stiffness, strength, and heat endurance.

The advancements in 2D titanium carbide MXene for tissue regeneration and other medical applications are thoroughly detailed in this chapter. This chapter is primarily concerned with Tin_1Cn, one of the most widely used titanium carbide MXenes. The essential scientific developments in 2D titanium carbide MXene and its applications are critically addressed. According to the needs and applications, this will provide an upgraded version of the latest scientific developments and studies to help readers comprehend and increase their interest in the possibilities of the newly developed 2D MXene for healthcare. This review chapter additionally emphasizes the useful idea of employing 2D titanium carbide MXene in various prospective applications. When tested and examined, the experimental findings showed good performance. Improvement in MXene and MXene family activity are also highlighted. The final section discusses future alterations to the newly discovered 2D titanium carbide MXene and highlights the conclusions and recommendations. Different properties and features of the emerging 2D MXene are illustrated in Table 7.1.

TABLE 7.1

Difference Properties and Features of the Emerging 2D MXenes

S. no.	Properties	Remarks	References
1.	**Mechanical properties**	Surface terminations have a substantial impact on the mechanical characteristics of MXenes. The materials with an O termination showed high stiffness, but those with OH terminations showed poor flexible stiffness. In particular, the surface-functionalized MXenes showed increased flexibility; the composite production based on MXene by using polym eric material of various kinds enhances the mechanical properties of MXenes, such as toughness, tensile, compressive, and flexibility	**[5]**
2.	**Electronic features**	The electronic properties of MXenes include semiconductivity, metallicity, topological insulative, and others. MXenes' conductivity is greatly influenced by the fabrication and exfoliation processes	**[5]**
3.	**Magnetic properties**	Many 2D materials are non-magnetic, which can restrict their use in spintronics. However, some MXenes, like Ti_2N, Cr_2C, and Ti_2C, are ferromagnetic, while others, like Cr_2N and Mn_2C, are antiferromagnetic, limiting their applicability in spintronics. MXenes' magnetic properties can be easily changed via surface functionalization	**[6]**
4.	**Optical properties**	It is possible to customize the MXene optical properties by modifying surface structural features. The properties of MXenes include a wide optical transparency window, non-linear visual performance, tunable optical response, strong plasmonic resonances, optical transmittance, and suitable photothermal transfer	**[7,19]**

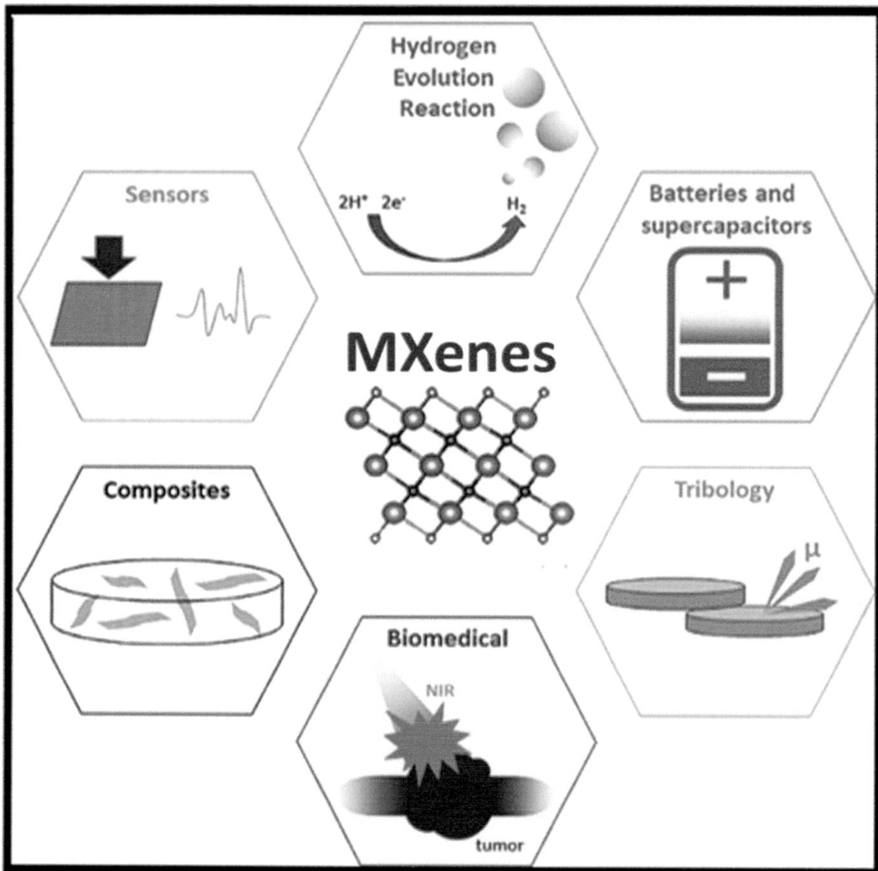

FIGURE 7.1
Structure and application of MXene [2].

As seen in Figure 7.1, MXene has many applications and uses in numerous areas. A series of 2D crystalline materials known as MXenes have atomically thin thicknesses and a potentially limitless diameter range. The characteristics of these materials vary from one another. Titanium carbide was the first MXene discovered (Ti_3C_2). It is employed in biological and environmental applications, including electromagnetic shielding, energy storage, and drinking water. The following are some common uses for MXene:

- In past recent years, MXene has been chiefly used as a filler material to create polymer composites.
- Due to its superior electronic properties, MXene material can be used in sensors that detect minute form variations.

- MXene has also decreased material microstructural changes and efficiently transferred tribofilm to the counter surface, improving tribological characteristics.
- MXene can be used in many biomedical sensor application, bioimaging, tissue engineering, and so on due to its unique 2D layered structure.

7.2 Structure and Synthesis of the Emerging 2D Titanium Carbide MXene

7.2.1 Structure of Titanium Carbide MXene

MXene is frequently used for medical and dental procedures, including implants and bone and spinal fixators. One newly researched material from the MXene family, with applications linked to energy and temperature, is titanium carbide (Ti_3C_2) [8]. Figure 7.2 illustrates how Ti_3C_2 can be employed for maximum charge holding in capacitance applications due to its layered electrochemically active surface. Additionally, it demonstrates remarkable and distinctive qualities such as metal-like conductivity for heat and electricity and ceramic qualities, including elastic stiffness, strength, and heat endurance. Ti and its alloys exert exceptional corrosion resistance and good hard-tissue compatibility.

7.2.2 Synthesis of Titanium Carbide MXene

Ti_3C_2 is a 2D transition metal carbide that belongs to the MXene class of two-dimensional transition metal carbides and nitrides, together with the initial

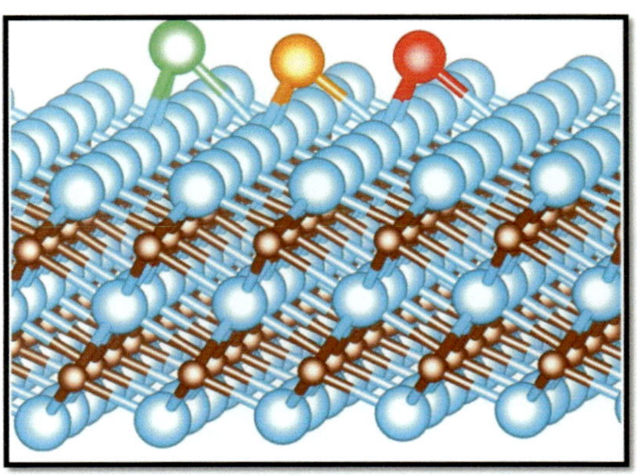

FIGURE 7.2
Structure of titanium carbide MXene [9].

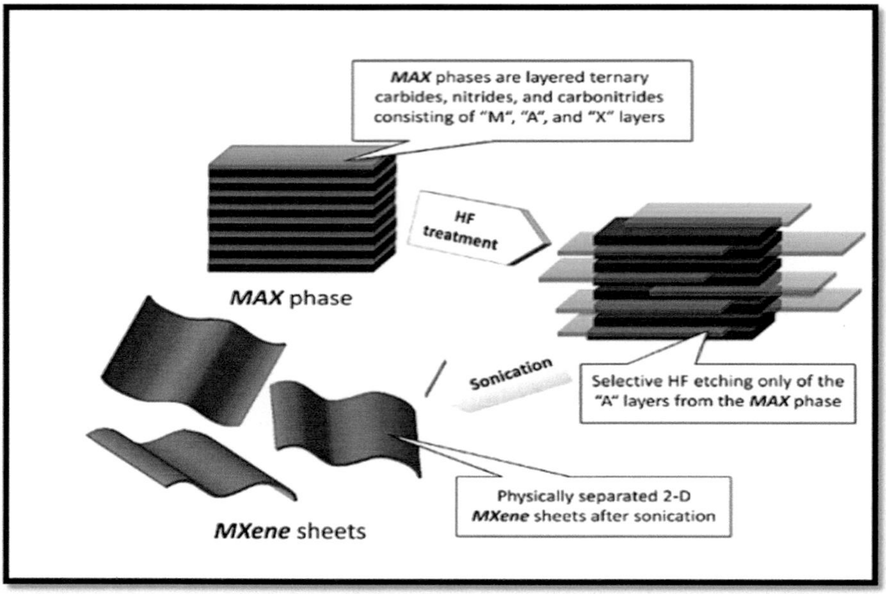

FIGURE 7.3
Synthesis of MAX phase to nanosheets of MXene [11].

transition metals Ti, V, Nb, and Mo. X can either be carbon or nitrogen [10]. Tin_1AlCn powder makes titanium carbide MXenes in their MAX phase. Tin_1AlCn powder is created by the powders of TiC, Ti, and Al, and activates carbon. Precursors should be in the MAX phase and ball-milled in 100% alcohol for 24 hours before being used to create MAX powder. Powders that have been blended are sieved and then vacuum-dried. Then, these powders are heated in a flowing argon environment. Then, they can be exfoliated by dipping the manufactured particles into hydrofluoric acid (HF) at room temperature. Etching is a crucial step in creating functional groups that are adhered to the surfaces of the MXenes, as shown in Figure 7.3.

7.3 Tissue Regeneration

Renewal and growth, known as tissue regeneration, are used to treat or replace diseased or damaged tissue [12]. In the human body, stem cells produce, maintain, and replenish tissues. In the human body, these specialized cells can develop into several cell types and undergo cell renewal since stem cells contain several differentiation pathways; they can differentiate into any form of body cell or a particular cell type with a specific function. For

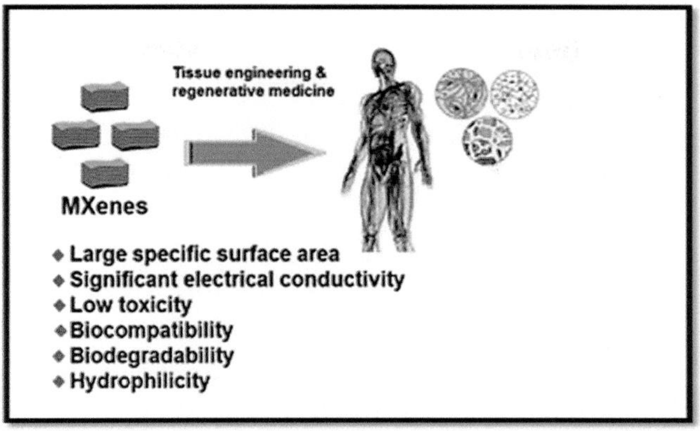

FIGURE 7.4
Properties of MXene [5].

biological applications and regenerative medicine, stem cells are increasingly the preferred molecular instrument due to their amazing potential for various functions. The high hydrophobicity, chemical stability, heat capacity, sorption selectivity, biocompatibility, and antimicrobial activities of MXenes and MXene-based materials, in contrast to these 2D materials, make them appealing candidates for tissue engineering, as displayed in Figure 7.4. Thus, it makes MXene preferable for tissue engineering.

7.4 Emerging 2D Titanium Carbide MXene in Tissue Engineering for Healthcare Applications

The many different MXene compositions offer a suitable environment for property tuning and comprehending the connections between method, structure, and property. They possess an outstanding and distinctive quality that makes it possible to use them for tissue regeneration. Because of their mechanical and electrical similarities to other two-dimensional nanostructured materials including metal oxides, graphene, and boron nitride, MXene could replace other 2D materials in various applications. Here, we describe a collection of papers from various academics and scientists on using 2D titanium carbide MXene in tissue engineering and other medical applications.

For instance, Chuang et al. [13] carefully assembled (2D) Nb_2C MXene nanosheets (NSs) in conjunction with medical titanium plate (TP) implants to create a biofunctional Nb_2C@TP (NTP) therapeutic platform capable of multimodal infection control, including the ability to clear germs and regenerate tissue, as shown in Figure 7.5. In bulk, MAX-phase Nb_2AlC ceramics

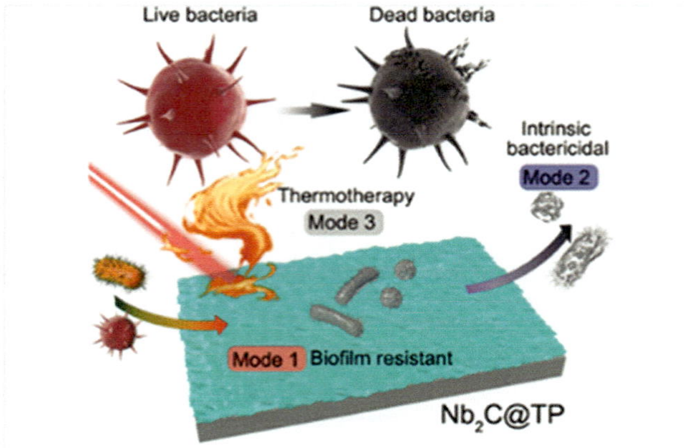

FIGURE 7.5
Graphical visualization of Nb_2C@TP's in vivo tissue renewal properties and trimodal bacterial killing strategy [13].

were etched with HF and exfoliated with tetrapropylammonium hydroxide (TPAOH) to yield Nb_2C NSs. Next, Nb_2C@TP was created by grafting Nb2C NSs onto amidated TPs (TPs-NH2) via electrostatic interactions. Nb_2C@TP is essential for the multimodal suppression of bacteria. Regarding the removal of biofilms, Nb_2C@TP triggers the activation of the accessory gene regulator (Agr) in response to bacterial invasion of the implant surface, thereby impeding bacterial adhesion and facilitating biofilm separation. Additionally, Nb_2C@TP directly killed bacteria by downregulating metabolic pathways like the PTS pathway and the tricarboxylic acid (TCA) cycle. Nb_2C@TP sensitized bacteria to hyperthermia and killed bacteria using NIR-responsive thermotherapy regarding planktonic bacterial clearance. Nb_2C@TP not only had a high ability to remove bacteria but also reduced oxidative stress and excessive proinflammatory responses in vivo, which sped up angiogenesis and the process of tissue remodeling. Notably, with its dual capabilities of tissue remodeling and bacterial/biofilm clearing, the thoughtfully designed multifunctional Nb_2C@TP offers hope for infections associated with implants [13].

For heart tissue engineering applications, Basara et al. created a unique composite construct that could provide topographical and conductive signals to human induced pluripotent stem cell-generated cardiomyocytes (iCMs) [14]. The constructs are created by employing aerosol jet printing to 3D print conductive titanium carbide ($Ti_3C_2T_x$) MXene in pre-planned patterns on polyethylene glycol (PEG) hydrogels at a cell-level resolution. The constructs are then seeded with iCMs and grown for a week without exhibiting cytotoxic effects. The results demonstrate how important 3D-printed $Ti_3C_2T_x$ MXene is for aligning iCMs with better synchronous beating and conduction velocity

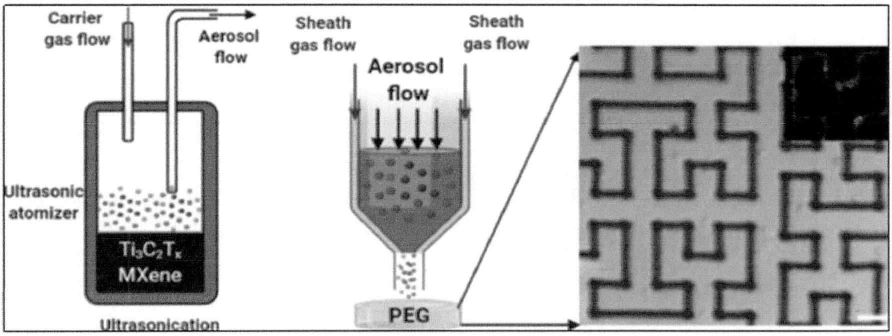

FIGURE 7.6
Fabrication of the construct by aerosol jet printing to 3D print conductive titanium carbide ($Ti_3C_2T_x$) [14].

and a considerable rise in MYH7, SERCA2, and TNNT2 expressions. To cure myocardial infarction (MI), this study shows that physiologically suitable cardiac patches made of 3D printed $Ti_3C_2T_x$ MXene may be possible (Figure 7.6).

Tianhui et al. developed novel composites consisting of $Ti_3C_2T_x$ nanosheets, with PDA, and biologically inert SCFPEEK. These components provide the bio-inert composites with two distinct therapeutic features: in vivo osseointegration and photothermal antibacterial activity. To the best of their knowledge, this was the first demonstration of a CFPEEK implant with a bioactive surface altered by $Ti_3C_2T_x$ nanosheets [15]. When $Ti_3C_2T_x$ and PDA were treated with synergistic photothermal therapy (PTT), the temperature rose to 40.8–59.6°C (SCP-PDA-Ti) as a result of heat absorption by SCFPEEK-PDA-$Ti_3C_2T_x$ (SCP-PDA-Ti). This high temperature caused bacterial death. After 10 minutes of near-infrared (NIR) irradiation at 808 nm, the SCP-PDA-Ti materials could successfully kill bacteria. A 100% bacteriostasis rate was attained by SCP-PDA-Ti (2.5) and SCP-PDA-Ti (3.0). More importantly, the multifaceted implant SCP-PDA-Ti shows strong cytocompatibility and a remarkable ability to induce bone formation in terms of diffusion, real-time PCR evaluation, alkaline phosphatase activity, and in vivo bone defect bone formation tests. This offers a more flexible development concept for orthopedic implant applications, including carbon fiber-reinforced composites.

Collagen type I and 2D MXenes ($Ti_3C_2T_x$) were combined in the work of Asaro et al. to create conductive biohybrid platforms, which were then covalently cross-linked to maximize the protein portion biofunctionality and the improved rigorousness and electrical conductivity that two-dimensional titanium carbide offers [16]. When fibroblasts were planted onto these highly biocompatible MXene platforms, the outcome was enhanced proliferation and cell spreading. On the other hand, they restricted the attachment and growth of *Staphylococcus aureus* bacteria.

Compared to control collagen substrates, enhanced spreading and viability were seen when neonatal rat cardiomyocytes (nrCMs) were grown on the substrates until day 7. In a specially designed bioreactor, electric-field production was used to seed and activate human induced pluripotent stem cell-derived cardiomyocytes (iPSC-CMs). An external electrical field and an electroconductive substrate combined greatly boosted cx43 expression and improved cell development. This compellingly illustrates the promise of this designed conducting biohybrid platform for heart tissue regeneration in an in vitro investigation.

7.5 Fabrication of Composite Nanofibers

Ti_3AlC_2 and LiF were mixed with HCl solution to create MXene nanosheets, which were then treated by centrifuging the solid residue after repeatedly rinsing it with DI water. DI water was added to the resultant solid residue and then held for sonication in an argon atmosphere. The resultant suspension was centrifuged to obtain the delaminated MXene nanosheets. Second, MXene nanosheets were combined with DCM and DMF to disperse them. After the dispersion had been sonicated, the prepared solution was stirred while PLLA and PHA were added. Third, an electrospun syringe was filled with the combined solution. Nanofibers made of MXene composite were manufactured and gathered as a result. Model cells called BMSCs were employed to examine the response to composite nanofibers of MXene, and the control groups used PLLA-PHA nanofibers. The surface of the manufactured composite nanofibers was shown to be smooth. In cooperation with PHA-PLLA nanofibers, the composite nanofibers' diameter distribution was worse (i.e., the surface texture of the composite nanofiber became rough). The cell test results showed that the developed MXene composite nanofibers had excellent biocompatibility and significantly increased cellular activity. These composite nanofibers facilitated the transformation of BMSCs into osteoblasts. MXene is a new class of biomaterials with the potential to bridge the translational gap between materials engineering and stem cell-based tissue therapies as well as upcoming multi-task biomedical therapies. This is due to its superior biocompatibility and nano-effect.

Rafieerad et al. discussed the first applications of autofluorescent MXene quantum of Ti_3C_2 titanium carbide dots for 3D tissue engineering, immune modulation, and stem cell survival. In order to construct a 3D platform with better physicochemical qualities for stem cell distribution along with tissue repair, Ti_3C_2 MQDs are added to a hydrogel based on chitosan. This hybrid hydrogel keeps its injection capability and thermosensitivity while exhibiting enhanced conductivity. SEM, TEM, EDS, and FTIR studies on the hydration properties, microbial degradation, and conduction of as-synthesized CS-MQD hydrogels were used to evaluate their structural and physicochemical characteristics. These results suggest that these distinct biomaterials may overcome the translational hurdle in stem cell and material-based therapies for tissue repair and treating inflammatory and degenerative diseases [17].

Recent research has shown that ultrathin titanium carbide (Ti_3C_2) nanosheets can transform light energy into heat, making them ideal for tumor photothermal treatment (PTT). Researchers disclosed the development of superparamagnetic 2D Ti_3C_2 MXenes for extremely effective cancer theranostics. A specific MXene surface chemistry for the in situ production of superparamagnetic Fe_3O_4 nanocrystals on the exterior surface of Ti_3C_2 MXenes was used. Other studies have revealed that 2D Ti_3C_2 MXenes might be created for biosensing, fluorescence imaging, and antibacterial protection applications [18,20]. This has opened up a new study area for MXenes' potential uses in biomedicine. In this chapter, there is a description of a superparamagnetic Ti_3C_2 composite MXene utilized for MRI-guided PTT against cancer. These intricately built magnetic Ti_3C_2-based composite MXenes have high biocompatibility, ensuring their potential therapeutic application. Based on the different surface chemistry of MXenes, this work gives space for new opportunities to work under the functionalization of 2D nanosheets made of MXenes.

7.6 Conclusion

The role and application of the newly developed 2D-titanium carbide MXene in tissue engineering and its specialization in healthcare applications have been thoroughly summarized in this chapter. We have emphasized the 2D MXene's most recent developments and advancements. MXene and 2D titanium carbide MXene have been the subject of a separate section. To provide the MXene in use for the healthcare sector, various researchers have conducted several tests and research on the 2D titanium carbide MXene. According to studies, titanium carbide MXene, the first developed MXene, has a high regeneration rate. Numerous studies have revealed that the tissue regeneration activities of titanium carbide MXene provided remarkable results. All titanium MXene characteristics were created to maximize its use in all areas. According to various publications on the multi-functionalization of MXenes, the properties of titanium carbide in the medical field access and significantly widen the utilization and potential avenues of MXene-based 2D materials, particularly in tissue engineering and tissue regeneration technology and other specialized applications. In other words, MXene is an encouraging new two-dimensional nanomaterial with numerous industrial uses because of its high surface-to-volume ratio, distinctive surface structure, and practicable surface functionalization. As reported, titanium carbide MXene (Ti_3C_2) is a biomaterial with significant potential to bridge the gap between materials engineering, stem cell-based tissue therapies, and forthcoming biomedical therapies. Ti_3C_2Tx has a fully functionalized surface, making it simple to interact with other materials and dissolve in solvents. 2D titanium carbide MXene, a new category of biomaterial, has developed and changed due to numerous factors that allow its employment in tissue engineering for clinical purposes.

7.7 Future Perspectives

The exposure of 2D MXenes has dramatically expanded the variety of 2D materials and their possible applications. The work of MXene in numerous fields opens up many avenues for the multifunctionalization of two-dimensional MXenes by combining various functional components. The study's results suggest that MXene is perfect for enhancing the promising future of this scientific field. Advances in biomedicine and disease therapy have exploded with the introduction of 2D materials. Numerous investigations into the properties of MXene are being conducted to discover more its intriguing properties for potential applications in tissue regeneration.

Some points of recommendation may include:

- It is necessary to investigate new, environmentally friendly, and sustainable synthetic fabrication techniques for MXenes and ways to modify them for functional cutting-edge tissue engineering applications.
- The performance, stability, bioavailability, biodegradability, and biocompatibility of a substance can be improved with the help of appropriate biofunctionalization and chemical surface modifications. It also reduces negative side effects or immune system reactions and improves the substance's targeting ability.
- It is imperative to determine how MXenes' size and composition affect their properties and to examine how MXenes interact with cells.
- Systematic and analytical evaluation of toxic effects, biodegradability, biocompatibility, and biosafety issues are required.

References

1. Verma S, Dwivedi U, Chaturvedi K, Kumari N, Dhangar M, Hashmi SA, Singhal R, Srivastava AK. Progress of 2D MXenes based composites for

efficient electromagnetic interference shielding applications: A review. Synthetic Metals 2022 Jul 1;287:117095.

2. RM Ronchi, JT Arantes, SF Santos. Synthesis, structure, properties and applications of MXenes: Current status and perspectives. Ceramics International 2019; 45(15):18167–18188. S0272884219316153. https://doi.org/10.1016/j.ceramint.2019.06.114
3. Chaturvedi K, Hada V, Paul S, Sarma B, Malvi D, Dhangar M, Bajpai H, Singhwane A, Srivastava AK, Verma S. The rise of MXene: A wonder 2D material, from its synthesis and properties to its versatile applications—A comprehensive review. Topics in Current Chemistry 2023 Mar;381(2):11.
4. Singhwane A, Chaturvedi K, Mohapatra RK, Srivastava AK, Verma S. Mxene-Based Composite Materials as Antibacterial Agents for Healthcare Applications. In Age of MXenes, Volume 2. Applications in Diagnostics, Therapeutics, and Environmental Remediation 2023. American Chemical Society, 2023, pp. 1–17.
5. Iravani S, Varma RS. MXenes and MXene-based materials for tissue engineering and regenerative medicine: Recent advances. Materials Advances 2021. 2(9):2906-2917. https://doi.org/10.1039/d1ma00189b
6. Han M, Maleski K, Shuck CE, Yang Y, Glazar JT, Foucher AC, Hantanasirisakul K, Sarycheva A, Frey NC, May SJ, Shenoy VB, Stach EA, Gogotsi Y. Tailoring electronic and optical properties of MXenes through forming solid solutions. Journal of the American Chemical Society 2020;142:19110–19118.
7. Wu Q, Chen S, Wang Y, Wu L, Jiang X, Zhang F, Jin X, Jiang Q, Zheng Z, Li J, Zhang M, Zhang H. MZI-based all-optical modulator using MXene Ti3C2Tx (T= F, O, or OH) deposited microfiber. Advanced Materials Technologies 2019;4:1800532.
8. Syamsai R, Kollu P, Kwan Jeong S, Nirmala Grace A. Synthesis and properties of 2D-Titanium carbide MXene sheets towards electrochemical energy storage applications. Ceramics International 2017;43(16):13119–13126. S0272884217314177. https://doi.org/10.1016/j.ceramint.2017.07.003
9. Gao Y, Cao Y, Gu Y, Zhuo H, Zhuang G, Deng S, Zhong X, Wei Z, Chen J, Pan X, Wang J-g. Functionalization Ti_3C_2 MXene by the adsorption or substitution of single metal atom. Applied Surface Science 2019;465:911–918. https://doi.org/10.1016/j.apsusc.2018.09.254
10. Feng AH, Yu Y, Wang Y, et al. Two-dimensional MXene Ti_3C_2 produced by exfoliation of Ti_3AlC_2. Materials & Design 2017;114:161–166.
11. Naguib M, Mashtalir O, Carle J, Presser V, Lu J, Hultman L, Gogotsi Y, Barsoum MW. Two-dimensional transition metal carbides. American Chemical Society Nano 2012;6(2):1322–1331.
12. Kaoud HA El-S. Introductory chapter: Concepts of tissue regeneration. In Tissue Regeneration. (Chapter 1), Intechopen. 2018. https://doi.org/10.5772/intechopen.76996
13. Yang C, Luo Y, Lin H, Ge M, Shi J, Zhang X. Niobium carbide MXene augmented medical implant elicits bacterial infection elimination and tissue regeneration. American Chemical Society Nano 2020;15(1):1086–1099. https://doi.org/10.1021/acsnano.0c08045
14. Basara G, Saeidi-Javash M, Ren X, Bahcecioglu G, Wyatt BC, Anasori B, Zhang Y, Zorlutuna P. Electrically conductive 3D printed $Ti_3C_2T_x$ MXene-PEG

composite constructs for cardiac tissue engineering. Acta Biomaterialia 2020;139:179–189.

15. Du T, Zhao S, Dong W, Ma W, Zhou X, Wang Y, Zhang M. Surface modification of carbon fiber-reinforced polyetheretherketone with MXene nanosheets for enhanced photothermal antibacterial activity and osteogenicity. ACS Biomaterials Science & Engineering 2022;8(6):2375–2389. https://doi.org/10.1021/acsbiomaterials.2c00095
16. Asaro GA, Solazzo M, Suku M., et al. MXene functionalized collagen biomaterials for cardiac tissue engineering driving iPSC-derived cardiomyocyte maturation. NPJ 2D Materials and Applications 2023; 7:44. https://doi.org/10.1038/s41699-023-00409-w
17. Rafieerad A, Yan W, Sequiera GL, Sareen N, Abu-El-Rub E, Moudgil M, Dhingra S. Application of Ti_3C_2 MXene quantum dots for immunomodulation and regenerative medicine. Advanced Healthcare Materials 2019; 8(16):1900569. https://doi.org/10.1002/adhm.201900569
18. Liu Z, Zhao M-L, Lin H, Chen D, Ren C-Y, Zhang S, Peng W, Chen Y. 2D Magnetic titanium carbide (MXene) for cancer theranostics. Journal of Materials Chemistry B 2018;6:3541–3548. https://doi.org/10.1039/C8TB00754C
19. Michael J, Qifeng Z, Danling W. Titanium carbide MXene: Synthesis, electrical and optical properties and their applications in sensors and energy storage devices. Nanomaterials and Nanotechnology 2019;9:184798041882447. https://doi.org/10.1177/1847980418824470
20. Li ZY, Wang LB, Sun DD, et al. Synthesis and thermal stability of two-dimensional carbide MXene Ti_3C_2. Materials Science and Engineering B Advances 2015;191:33–40.

8

MXene-Based 'Therapeutic Agents'

Gagan Kant Tripathi, Shikha Katre, Pradeep Khiriya, Priyavand Bundela, Purnima Swarup Khare, and Priyanka Dixit

8.1 Introduction

Therapeutics and medicines, generally described as remedial agents, are composites employed to address, palliate, or cure numerous medical conditions and diseases. They can be administered through intravenous infusions, topical creams, injections, or orally ingested tablets. These substances ply their goods through different mechanisms, such as modifying physiological processes, reducing the intensity of symptoms, or targeting specific chemical pathways. Certain remedial agents bind to specific receptors within the body, while others may stymie the product of particular enzymes. The ultimate ideal of these remedial agents is to restore, maintain, or cure the body's normal functioning, thereby enhancing overall health. Exemplifications of typical remedial agent orders include antibiotics, anesthetics, antiviral agents, antidepressants, antiinflammatory agents, antitumor agents, anticancer agents, and more.

Antibiotics specifically target bacteria. They work by either killing the bacteria or precluding their growth. Common exemplifications of antibiotics include penicillin, amoxicillin, and tetracycline [1]. Healthcare professionals specify these specifics to treat infections, such as urinary tract infections, respiratory infections, and skin infections. Anesthetics are generally used to relieve mild to moderate pain, like headaches, muscle pangs, and menstrual cramps. They work by reducing inflammation and blocking pain signals in the body. They include acetaminophen and ibuprofen [2]. Antiviral rectifiers are used to palliate viral infections similar to influenza or HIV. They work by inhibiting the replication of contagions and reducing the inflexibility and duration of symptoms. They can be used for treatment to combat viral infections effectively [3–5]. Antidepressants are the drugs administered to treat depression and mood diseases, and include sertraline and fluoxetine, to help regulate neurotransmitters in the brain and improve

DOI: 10.1201/9781003353287-8

symptoms of depression [6,7]. Antiinflammatory agents are pivotal in managing conditions such as arthritis and asthma. These medications, which include corticosteroids, help in lowering inflammation [8,9]. Antineoplastic rectifier agents are a family of medicines used especially to prevent cancer cells from proliferating and spreading [10]. As an example, cisplatin is frequently employed in the treatment of several cancer types, including testicular, ovarian, and bladder cancers [11]. Tamoxifen, on the other hand, is frequently recommended for cases with hormone receptor-positive bone cancer in order to stymie the excrescence's proliferation or rush [12]. Antihypertensive medicines are used to rehabilitate and lower the blood pressure. These medicines efficiently lowering blood pressure by depressing blood arterials and reducing the heart's strain. In order to gain the required consequences in restraining hypertension, they are constantly bestowed in confluence with life variations, including a nutritional diet and harmonious exercise [13]. Anticoagulants are medicines used to prevent blood clots from forming, such as warfarin. This has a particular risk drift for those who are endangered by blood clots, such as those who have a history of deep vein thrombosis or atrial fibrillation. Anticoagulants help maintain blood flow and reduce the risk of life-threatening side effects including stroke or pulmonary embolism. To guarantee the drug's efficacy and avoid any side effects, blood-clotting agents must be regularly monitored [14]. Insulin and metformin, two antidiabetic medications, are employed to treat diabetes. Metformin is frequently used as the first line of treatment for type 2 diabetes due to its demonstrated ability to decrease blood sugar levels and improve insulin sensitivity. Once again, in more severe forms of diabetes, insulin is always used when conventional medications are unable to effectively control blood sugar levels [15,16]. Immunosuppressants are medications used by patients undergoing organ transplants or those repeatedly suffering from autoimmune diseases to weaken their susceptible systems. They contain ingredients comparable to cyclosporine. These medications work by preventing susceptible cells requesting help, which prevents them from attacking organ transplant recipients. Immunosuppressants can increase the risk of infections and other side effects over time, therefore situations involving these must be carefully managed and completely covered [17]. Since synchronous medications provide a wide range of cures for various medical afflictions, restorative actions are required.

These medicinal drugs can treat chronic illnesses, alleviate symptoms, and even cure them, thereby greatly improving the patient's quality of life. Pharmaceutical patronage continues to improve drugs through intense research, development, and testing, leading to more precise treatments with fewer side effects. Therefore, it is necessary to bear in mind that strict regulation, administration, and meticulous use are necessary for the protection and effectiveness of therapeutic medications. Investigating novel and personalized medications could result in more effective results with reduced patient problems [18]. Nanomaterial-based therapeutics is a novel approach in the medical and healthcare fields. These cutting-edge tools, which are often nanoscale, have unique capabilities and calibers that have the potential to completely transform the treatment of a variety of illnesses. Using nanotechnology, scientists and researchers have produced nanoparticles and nanocarriers that can transport drugs or other restorative substances with previously unheard of rigor. Drug effectiveness can be increased and adverse effects can be decreased by altering these nanomaterials to target specific cells or tissues.

Additionally, they can improve the solubility and hardness of poorly soluble medications, making them more suitable for clinical use. Nanomaterial-based treatments show promise in gene therapy, cancer treatment, and diagnostics, creating new opportunities for precise and customized medications. Curatives based on nanomaterials have the potential to change how we approach and treat a wide range of medical conditions as this field of research advances. Additionally, nanomaterial-based therapies can target unknown cells or tissues, increasing their effectiveness and reducing harm to healthy cells. This focused approach may result in improved treatment outcomes and reduced toxicity as compared to current therapeutics. Similarly, drugs can be designed to be released from nanomaterials in a controlled manner, enabling continuous drug delivery and possibly reducing the number of boluses that patients need to swallow [19,20].MXene nanosheets are a genre of two-dimensional materials that have recently received an enormous amount of interest across all areas of nanotechnology. These materials are an instance of transition metal carbide, nitride, or carbonitride, and are usually produced by selectively stripping the 'A' layer from MAX phases. MXene nanosheets possess high electrical conductivity, a high degree of mechanical strength, and a large surface area, making them a suitable option in a variety of applications, including energy storage, water purification, and electronic devices [21]. MXenes have additionally demonstrated suitability in several biomedical applications, including drug delivery, imaging, and tissue engineering [22]. MXenes provide a new direction for cutting-edge medical research because of their enormous potential as multifunctional materials for the creation of medicinal drugs and biomedical technologies [23]. Furthermore, MXenes have demonstrated encouraging outcomes in systems for drug delivery, where their substantial surface area facilitates effective loading and regulated release of medicinal substances. MXene nanosheets' unique mix of qualities and adaptability make them potential revolutionary developments in a number of sectors.

The uncontrolled growth and proliferation of aberrant cells inside the body is the hallmark of a complex and multifaceted group of disorders known as cancer. These cells have the potential to become tumors, disrupt regular body processes, and pose a serious risk to life if unchecked. Any region of the body can be affected by cancer, for several reasons, such as genetic abnormalities, exposure to toxins, and certain lifestyle choices [24]. For those with cancer, improving outcomes depends on early identification and prompt treatment.

There are several types of cancer, and each has a unique combination of symptoms and risk factors. Genetic mutations, environmental variables like tobacco use and UV radiation, and lifestyle decisions like nutrition and exercise are frequently blamed for the development of cancer. Several techniques, including imaging, biopsies, and blood testing, can be used to diagnose cancer. Treatment options may include immunotherapy, chemotherapy, radiation therapy, surgery, and targeted treatments, depending on a number of parameters, such as the particular type and stage of the cancer [25,26]. Cancer outcomes have greatly improved due to early identification and advancements in medical research, highlighting the need for routine screenings and a healthy lifestyle to lower the individual's risk.

The discovery and development of new antitumor drugs is vital for combating cancer. MXene nanosheets provide a viable delivery system for antitumor medications. We discuss how MXene nanosheets can be functionalized to precisely encapsulate and distribute therapeutic payloads to tumor sites. By using a customized medication-delivery strategy, antitumor therapies can be more effective and have fewer side effects. Researchers may attach specific targeted molecules that identify and bind to malignant cells by functionalizing MXene nanosheets. By doing this, the antitumor medications are guaranteed to reach the malignant cells directly, minimizing harm to healthy tissues and boosting the treatment's overall efficacy. MXene nanosheets show potential not just as antitumor agents but also as direct anticancer agents. Researchers have investigated how MXene nanosheets may hinder the development of tumors and cause the death of cancer cells [27,28]. To cause cancer cells to die, photothermal therapy (PTT), an emerging cancer treatment technique, uses targeted heating. The outstanding photothermal characteristics of MXene nanosheets make them ideal for PTT [29]. The potential of MXene nanosheets as photothermal agents and techniques for precision cancer cell targeting have been discussed. Chemotherapy remains a mainstay of cancer care. The usage of MXene nanosheets as chemotherapeutic medication carriers is carried out due to their capacity to lower systemic toxicity and improve medication delivery to cancer cells.

Innovative therapeutic agents can now be developed with intriguing prospects provided by the science of nanotechnology. MXene nanosheets and other nanomaterials have drawn much interest because of their special qualities, including large surface area, outstanding biocompatibility, and adjustable surface chemistry [27]. In this chapter, we examine MXene nanosheets' involvement in therapeutics, emphasizing their potential as antitumor and anticancer drugs. We also discuss how they may be used in photothermal therapy and chemotherapy, two promising approaches to treating cancer. MXene nanosheets have also demonstrated significant promise in targeted drug-delivery systems, enabling the exact and regulated release of therapeutic chemicals straight to cancer cells. Furthermore, they provide a viable option for combination therapy due to their capacity to increase the effectiveness of currently available chemotherapeutic medications through synergistic effects, making them a promising candidate for combination therapy approaches in cancer treatment.

8.2 Role of MXene Nanosheets in Therapeutics

Two-dimensional materials known as MXene nanosheets have drawn a lot of interest from a variety of industries, including in medicine. At Drexel University in Philadelphia, US, two teams led by Yury Gogotsi and Michel Barsoum discovered MXene in 2011. $M_{n+1}X_nT_x$ is the general formula for the thin layer of nitrides, carbides, or carbonitride of early transition metals. Here, M stands for early transition metals, such as Sc, Ti, Cr, V, Y, Zr, Nb, Mo, Hf, Ta, and W; n = 1–3 and denotes layers of transition metals; X stands for carbides, nitrides, or carbonitride; and T_x stands for surface transitions, such as O, F, Cl, and H. They created structures resembling laminates. When pure group elements (A) and X-atom-filled sites are interleaved between M (transition metal) layers, MAX phases can form MXene. On the other hand, etching the A-layers from the MAX phases allows for the synthesis of MXene [30]. MXene is renowned for bearing special qualities that lend themselves to potentially attractive options for various therapeutic applications.

8.2.1 Properties of MXene Nanosheets

Because of their special qualities and adaptability, MXene nanosheets have demonstrated potential in therapeutic applications. Among the essential characteristics of MXene nanosheets that render them useful for treatments are the following:

Biocompatibility: MXene nanosheets are biocompatible when altered or modified, meaning that when injected into living things, they do not trigger toxic effects or detrimental immune responses. They mimic tissue or cells. This attribute holds significance in terms of their utilization in therapeutics.

Surface functionalizations: Different functional groups and biomolecules can be attached to MXene nanosheets due to their adjustable surface chemistry. Their potential as drug carriers is increased by this trait, which allows tailored drug delivery.

High surface area: MXene nanosheets are excellent candidates to transport therapeutic agents like medicines or drugs, proteins, or nucleic acids because of their high surface area, which offers an adequate area to interact for drug loading.

Antimicrobial properties: Certain MXenes are reported to possess antimicrobial properties, making them potentially helpful in the battle against infections. To lower the risk of infection, they can be applied as coatings on medical equipment or included in wound dressings.

Electro-conductivity: The electrical conductivity of MXene nanosheets has potential benefits for specific medical uses. For instance, they can be included in conductive scaffolds for tissue engineering or utilized in electrostimulation treatments.

Biodegradability: Some MXene nanosheets can be made to be biodegradable, thereby reducing their subsequent presence in the body once therapy is finished, depending on the particular MXene composition and structure.

Itis crucial to remember that MXene nanosheet research for therapeutic uses is still in progress, and clinical settings may not be using these materials for therapeutic purposes. More research is required to prove their safety and usefulness for a range of therapeutic uses. MXene nanosheets have the potential to advance medication delivery, medical diagnostics, and therapeutics significantly (Figure 8.1).

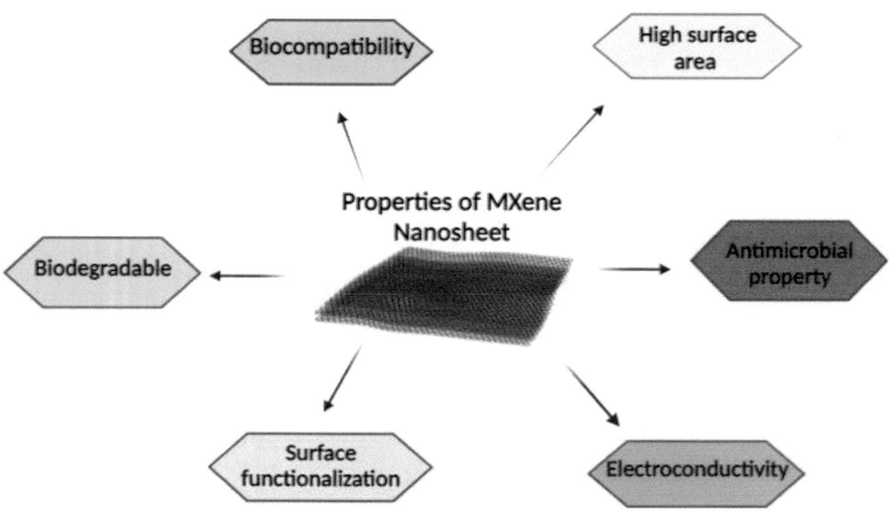

FIGURE 8.1
Properties of MXene nanosheets.

8.2.2 Roles and Potential Applications of MXene Nanosheets in Therapeutics

Drug delivery: Drugs can be delivered using MXene nanosheets. Because of their vast surface area and functionalization capacities, they may be used to load and distribute a wide range of therapeutic agents, including medications, proteins, and nucleic acids. They are useful for regulated drug-delivery systems because of their high loading capacity and capability to release pharmaceuticals in response to particular triggers such as pH, temperature, or enzymes. They can carry more drugs due to their large surface area and two-dimensional shape, promoting effective cellular absorption.

Photothermal therapy: Certain MXene nanosheets have significant photothermal characteristics, implying they effectively convert light energy into heat. They can produce heat when exposed to near-infrared light, which can be used in photothermal treatment to target and eliminate infections or cancer cells.

Imaging: MXene nanosheets can be functionalized with contrast or fluorescent dyes for fluorescence imaging, magnetic resonance imaging (MRI), and computed tomography (CT) scans. This makes it possible to monitor and observe the progress of therapy and medication distribution.

Combination therapies: To improve the overall effectiveness of treatment, MXene nanosheets can be utilized in conjunction with other therapeutic methods such as immunotherapy, radiation therapy, or chemotherapy.

Tissue regeneration: MXene nanosheets can be utilized in tissue engineering scaffolds to promote repairing injured or damaged tissues, especially in orthopedic applications, wound healing, and injury situations. They are helpful in regenerative medicine because of their mechanical strength, biocompatibility, and capacity to promote cell adhesion and proliferation.

Antibacterial agents: The antimicrobial qualities of MXene nanosheets may be used to create antibacterial coatings, bandages, and other materials that either avoid or mitigate infections caused by bacteria. Their unusual surface chemistry makes it possible for infections to engage directly with them or for antimicrobial drugs to adhere to them.

Biosensors: The development of biosensors for identifying certain biomolecules or disease indicators can use MXene nanosheets. Their excellent electrical conductivity and biocompatibility facilitate their ability to integrate with different biological recognition components, such as DNA probes or antibodies.

Neural interfaces: MXene nanosheets have shown promise in developing neural and brain–machine interfaces. Their electrical conductivity and

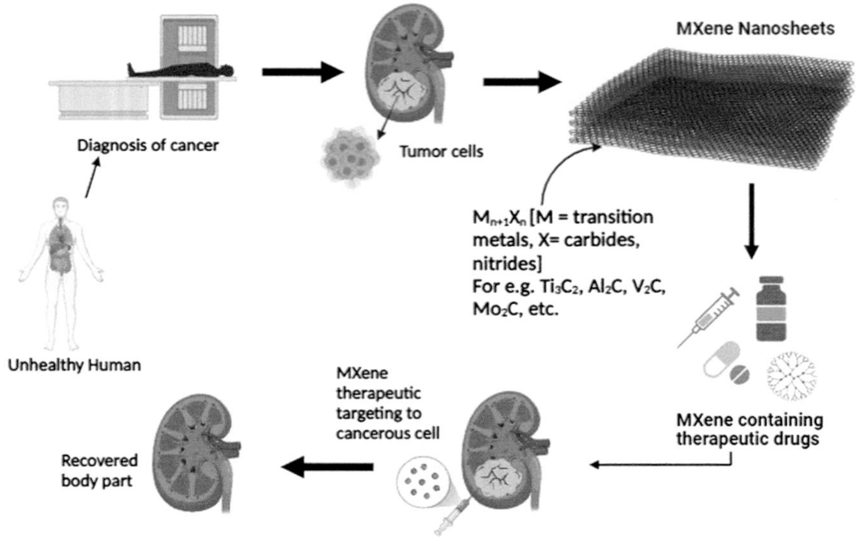

FIGURE 8.2
Role of MXenes as anticancer therapeutics.

biocompatibility make them suitable for transmitting electrical signals between neural tissue and external devices.

Anticancer treatment: Functionalized MXene nanosheets can release therapeutic chemicals and particularly target cancer cells in addition to medication delivery and photothermal treatment. Additionally, combination therapies can be employed with them, such as combining photothermal therapy with chemotherapeutic medications.

Antioxidant and antiinflammatory agents: MXene nanosheets have been studied for their potential in these capacities. They may be used to treat illnesses linked to oxidative stress and inflammation because of their ability to salvage free radicals and lower inflammation.

Itis crucial to remember that the stream of study on MXene nanosheets with therapeutics is still in its infancy and that every distinctive implementation requires a careful analysis of their reliability and efficacy. Nevertheless, they represent exciting materials for various therapeutic uses due to their special qualities and adaptability (Figure 8.2).

8.2.3 Antitumor Agents

Hao et al. concluded that MXene-based $Nb_2CPtDOX$ has a plasmonic complex of biocatalyst to treat tumors; where Nb_2C plasmon is MXene, Pt is nanozymes, and DOX is doxorubicin. They act as antitumor agents. Based on

MXene, they created a novel NIR-II triggered biomimetic plasmonic assembly for tumor treatment. MXene-based plasmonic technology allowed us to overcome the poor efficiency problem of most biomimetic nanocarriers. When the NPD@M was exposed to NIR-II laser light, charge density ridges of MXene and Pt nanozymes were collected and integrated into cancer cells, producing increased O_2 and ROS. The complex was able to reverse multidrug resistance by down-regulating HIF-1α and diminishing the mitochondrial energy supply for P-gp glycoprotein. In addition, it reinforced chemotherapy and worked in conjunction with tumor-penetrating photothermal treatment to enhance tumor regression. In summary, using plasmonic assembly to augment the activity of nanozymes in this investigation has expanded the potential uses of MXene for antitumor purposes. Additionally, it has established a novel paradigm for plasmonic assembly to enhance the activity of nanozymes, thereby contributing to the advancement of biocatalysis in tumor therapy [31,32].

In 2018, Liu and colleagues utilized magnetic MXenes for an effective approach to treating cancer. They harnessed the enhanced photothermal conversion capabilities of MXene to improve photothermal therapy (PTT) against cancer. Additionally, they employed iron oxide nanoparticles (IONPs) to serve as a contrast agent for T2-weight magnetic resonance imaging (MRI). To enhance the biocompatibility and stability of the MXene-IONPs in physiological conditions, they incorporated soybean phospholipids (Ti_3C_2-IONPs-SPs).In their experimental setup, they administered Ti_3C_2-IONPs-SPs via intravenous injection and subsequently exposed the tumor to near-infrared (NIR) laser radiation (1.5 Wcm^{-2}, 808 nm) for 8 minutes. An infrared thermal imaging camera was used to monitor the changes in tumor temperature. The group treated with laser + Ti_3C_2-IONPs-SPs experienced a rapid increase in tumor temperature following NIR laser irradiation, in contrast to the group treated with laser alone, which saw only a 2°C temperature rise. Remarkably, the tumor in the former group significantly regressed, leaving a dark scar at the tumor site during the initial days.

Conversely, the tumors in the other groups continued to grow over a 16-day observation period. Overall, this nanocomposite, Ti_3C_2-IONPs, exhibited a high T2 relaxation rate of 394.2 $mM^{-1}s^{-1}$, making it suitable for MRI with efficient tumor contrast. Furthermore, Ti_3C_2-IONPs demonstrated substantial photothermal conversion efficiencies (48.6%) for reducing tumor tissue and eliminating cancer cells in vitro and in vivo, using BALB/c nude and Kunming mice as models [33].

8.2.4 Anticancer Agents

Feng et al. explored the creation of innovative, responsive structures for precise drug delivery in cancer therapy. They created zeolitic imidazolate framework-8 (ZIF-8), known for its extensive and well-defined surface area, which was employed to encapsulate both DOX and MXene quantum dots

(MQDs). This resulted in the formation of MQD combined ZIF-8/DOX, which exhibited exceptional photothermal conversion efficiency and the ability to generate reactive oxygen species (ROS), thus enabling effective photothermal therapy and photodynamic therapy. Furthermore, DOX was incorporated into MQD combined ZIF-8 nanoparticles and released at a pH of 5.6. The multifunctional drug-delivery system of MQD combined ZIF-8, where Zn^{2+} acted as nucleation sites on MQD. MQD-combined ZIF-8 composites were formed in situ through a rapid reaction between Zn^{2+} and 2-MIM molecules. In this system, the anticancer drug DOX was encapsulated within MQD combined ZIF-8, with MQD serving as both a photothermal agent (PTA) and a photosensitizer (PS). This allowed for a combination of photodynamic therapy (PDT) and photothermal therapy (PTT), as NIR light energy was efficiently converted into thermal energy and ROS were generated when exposed to UV laser irradiation, effectively eradicating cancer cells. Additionally, DOX release was significantly enhanced in the tumor microenvironment. Consequently, using the MQD-combined ZIF-8/DOX nanocarrier could achieve a combined approach of chemotherapy and phototherapy for tumor treatment [34].

In 2022, Zhang and team introduced a Ti_3C_2 nanosheet-based bionic cascaded-enzyme nanoreactor for combined tumor enzyme dynamic therapy (EDT), phototherapy, and deoxygenation-activated chemotherapy. By chemically binding glucose oxidase (GOX) and chloroperoxidase (CPO) to Ti_3C_2 nanosheets and loading the deoxygenation-activated drug tirapazamine (TPZ), they created Ti_3C_2-GOX-CPO/TPZ (TGCT), which was encapsulated in cancer cell-derived membrane vesicles with elevated CD47 expression (meTGCT). meTGCT benefits from biomimetic camouflage and CD47 overexpression, enhancing immune escape and tumor targeting. GOX and CPO generate HClO within tumor cells for effective EDT, boosted by laser irradiation's accelerated enzymatic reactions and increased singlet oxygen ($^1O_2$) production. The local hypoxic environment, coupled with oxygen depletion from EDT, activates a deoxygenation-sensitive prodrug for chemotherapy. As a result, meTGCT achieves amplified synergistic therapeutic effects encompassing tumor phototherapy, EDT, and chemotherapy for effective tumor control. This intelligent cascaded-enzyme nanoreactor presents a promising avenue for comprehensive antitumor therapy [35].

8.2.5 Chemotherapy

In 2018, Xing et al. produced cellulose-based hydrogel nanoplatforms based on MXene Ti_3C_2 nanosheets and the anticancer medication DOX for cancer chemotherapy. The ensuing MXene/DOX-doped cellulose composite hydrogel exhibits a substantial capacity to load DOX, superior photothermal assets, and acceptable biocompatibility. Likewise, because the medication release rate correlated proactively with the photothermal impact, it was independently controlled. As a result, this innovative drug-dispensing method enabled a comprehensive and curative approach in the tumor models that successfully killed tumors and stopped them from recurring. With the ultimate goal of achieving successful adept research and clinical and translational applications of light-activated MXene/DOX-combined cellulose hydrogel, further research into safeguarding easy, affordable, and regulated synthesis techniques of superior MXene nanomaterials with significantly improved efficacy and fewer adverse effects is imperative. The study conducted uncovered the methods by which this ingenious hydrogel-type nanoplatform, based on MXene polymer, worked as a curative cancer treatment. These mechanisms could be extended to other 2D inorganic materials [36].

Cancer cells typically exhibit a heightened need for iron, which plays a crucial role in driving their rapid growth, tumor advancement, and spread to other body parts. This heightened dependence on iron makes regulating iron in the body an appealing target for potential cancer treatments. In a study by Xu and colleagues in 2022, they introduced a novel dual-therapeutic prodrug named DOXjade, designed for chemo-photothermal cancer therapy, which combines the benefits of the clinically approved iron-chelating drug deferasirox (ExJade) with the topoisomerase 2 inhibitor doxorubicin (DOX). When DOXjade is loaded onto ultrathin 2D Ti_3C_2 MXene nanosheets, it creates a construct known as Ti_3C_2-PVP-loaded DOXjade. This construct enables the iron-chelating and chemotherapeutic properties of DOXjade to be activated by light at the tumor site, while also generating a strong photothermal effect with photothermal conversion efficiencies of up to 40%. Detailed examinations of how this therapy works against tumors revealed that once activated, Ti_3C_2-PVP-loaded DOXjade induces apoptotic cell death and reduces the iron transferrin receptor (TfR) overexpression caused by iron depletion. The treatment also responds to the acidic conditions found in tumors, enhancing its iron-chelating, photothermal, and chemotherapeutic effects in laboratory settings and living organisms. The findings from this research suggest that an iron chelation-based phototherapy approach holds promise for cancer treatment [37].

8.2.6 Photothermal Therapy

In 2019, Hussein and his team developed plasmonic nanocomposites, Au/Fe_3O_4/Ti_3C_2 and Au/Ti_3C_2, for anticancer photothermal therapy (PTT), which exhibited lower in vivo toxicity compared to Ti_3C_2. They evaluated the photothermal efficacy of Au/Fe_3O_4/MXene and Au/MXene on breast cancer cells (MCF7) after incubation with different nanocomposite concentrations, observing no cytotoxicity without laser exposure, demonstrating their high biocompatibility. Upon exposure to a NIR laser (808 nm, 1.0 W/cm^2) for 5 minutes, cell viability progressively decreased with increasing nanocomposite concentration. As a result, these new nanocomposites appear to be more suitable and safer than Ti_3C_2 for biomedical applications, particularly in PTT [38].

From bulk Nb_2C (BNC), a chemical exfoliation technique synthesized few-layered Nb_2C (FNC). It exhibited remarkable efficacy in diminishing ROS levels as per density functional theory (DFT) and demonstrated the ability to inhibit oxidative stress in invitro experiments. During the initial phases of osteoclast differentiation, ROS plays a crucial role in promoting the formation of osteoclasts. FNC effectively impeded osteoclast development by scavenging ROS and mitigating the associated signaling pathways. Furthermore, FNC treatment alleviated UHMWPE-induced osteolysis. With its antioxidant characteristics, FNC can reduce cytokine production and hinder osteoclastogenesis by adsorbing ROS. Additionally, in the mouse calvarial model, injecting FNC reduced UHMWPE-induced osteolysis. FNC holds promise for the treatment of osteolytic bone disorders arising from osteoclastogenesis [39].

Because of their substantial drug-loading ability, numerous drug-dispersion modalities, and superior biocompatibility, conveniently surface-modified MXenes have been widely explored as nanoplatforms enabling drug delivery. Researchers presented the creation of an MXene-blended Au-PEG drug-delivery mechanism that offers near-infrared (NIR) laser-triggered and pH-responsive drug release regimens for chemotherapeutic doxorubicin (DOX). The MXene-blended Au-PEG-DOX system exhibits high photothermal stability, biological safety, and histocompatibility during in vivo and in vitro experiments due to surface modification using thiol polyethylene glycol aldehyde chains (SH-PEG-CHO) coupled to the MXene by Au nanoparticles (Au NPs). Furthermore, due to the remarkable photothermal conversion capacity provided by both Au particles and MXene, the system demonstrates combinatorial photothermal blistering and chemotherapy as a tumor treatment. The MXene-blended Au-PEG drug-delivery platform enhances the controlled release of drugs, which, in turn, enhances the uptake of DOX by cells in tumor sites, ultimately boosting the effectiveness of the medication. Consequently, the suggested method for creating a surface-modified MXene-based drug-delivery platform, with a substantial drug-carrying capacity and various drug-release mechanisms, showcases a promising example of the potential use of MXene-based nanomaterials in treating cancer [40].

MXene, a two-dimensional (2D) vanadium carbide (V_2C) compound, has demonstrated tremendous promise as a photothermal agent (PTA) for photothermal treatment (PTT). However, the strict synthesis conditions and low photothermal conversion efficiency (PTCE) restrict the usage of V_2C in PTT. Systemic in vitro and in vivo investigations show that V_2C NSs can function as an effective PTA for photoacoustic (PA) and magnetic resonance imaging (MRI)-guided PTT of malignancy. This study presents a cost-effective, environmentally friendly, and high-yielding MAX disassembling method, opening up a new route for developing MXenes with desirable characteristics for various applications [41].

8.3 Conclusion

To summarize, the use of MXene nanosheets as therapeutic agents is a potential opportunity in the realm of medicine. MXene's unique features, such as large surface area, good conductivity, and biocompatibility, make it well-suited for various biomedical applications. Recent research has shown that MXene nanosheets have tremendous promise as drug-delivery vehicles, imaging agents, and even components in biosensors. Their capacity to interact at the nanoscale with biological systems opens up new avenues for targeted and customized therapeutics. Furthermore, because MXene nanosheets are programmable, their physicochemical features may be tailored to match specific therapeutic needs. While more research is needed to fully understand the long-term effects and potential challenges of using MXene in a therapeutic context, the current research indicates that MXene nanosheets hold great promise in advancing the development of innovative and effective medical interventions. MXene nanosheets have emerged as a valuable tool in this multidisciplinary field, opening the way for the next generation of therapeutic techniques as the junction of nanotechnology and medicine continues to expand.

References

1. Hutchings, Matthew I., Andrew W. Truman, and Barrie Wilkinson. "Antibiotics: Past, present and future." Current Opinion in Microbiology 51 (2019): 72–80.
2. Sharma, Archi. "Various biological activities of DHA derivatives." In Dehydroacetic Acid and its Derivatives, Elsevier, 2017, pp. 81–118.
3. Dhara, Amal Kumar, and Amit Kumar Nayak. "Introduction to antiviral therapy."(2023):3–22. Elsevier, www.sciencedirect.com/science/article/abs/pii/B9780323918145000258
4. Yang, Priscilla L. "Antiviral therapeutics." ACS Infectious Diseases 7, no. 6 (2021): 1297–1297.
5. Tompa, Dharma Rao, Aruldoss Immanuel, Srimari Srikanth, and Saraboji Kadhirvel. "Trends and strategies to combat viral infections: A review on FDA approved antiviral drugs." International Journal of Biological Macromolecules 172 (2021): 524–541.
6. Luo, Yan, Yuki Kataoka, Edoardo G. Ostinelli, Andrea Cipriani, and Toshi A. Furukawa. "National prescription patterns of antidepressants in the treatment of adults with major depression in the US between 1996 and 2015: A population representative survey based analysis." Frontiers in Psychiatry 11 (2020): 35.
7. Schechter, Lee E., Robert H. Ring, Chad E. Beyer, Zoë A. Hughes, Xavier Khawaja, Jessica E. Malberg, and Sharon Rosenzweig-Lipson. "Innovative

approaches for the development of antidepressant drugs: Current and future strategies." NeuroRx 2, no. 4 (2005): 590–611.
8. Mastalerz, Lucyna, and Hanna Kasperkiewicz. "Effect of inhaled corticosteroids on small airway inflammation in patients with bronchial asthma." Polish Archives of Internal Medicine 121, no. 7-8 (2011).
9. Dinarello, Charles A. "Anti-inflammatory agents: Present and future." Cell 140, no. 6 (2010): 935–950.
10. Wei, Guoxu, Min Wu, He Zhu, Sheng Han, Jing Chen, Chenchen Zhai, and Luwen Shi. "Off-label use of antineoplastic drugs to treat malignancies: Evidence from China based on a nationwide medical insurance data analysis." Frontiers in Pharmacology 12 (2021): 616453.
11. Dasari, Shaloam, and Paul Bernard Tchounwou. "Cisplatin in cancer therapy: Molecular mechanisms of action." European Journal of Pharmacology 740 (2014): 364–378.
12. Jordan, V. Craig. "Tamoxifen: A most unlikely pioneering medicine." Nature Reviews Drug Discovery 2, no. 3 (2003): 205–213.
13. Laurent, Stéphane. "Antihypertensive drugs." Pharmacological Research 124 (2017): 116–125.
14. Weitz, Jeffrey I. "New anticoagulant drugs." Journal of Thrombosis and Thrombolysis 12 (2001): 7–17.
15. Stein, Stephanie Aleskow, Elizabeth Mary Lamos, and Stephen N. Davis. "A review of the efficacy and safety of oral antidiabetic drugs." Expert Opinion on Drug Safety 12, no. 2 (2013): 153–175.
16. Wróbel, Marta Patrycja, Bogdan Marek, Dariusz Kajdaniuk, Dominika Rokicka, Aleksandra Szymborska-Kajanek, and Krzysztof Strojek. "Metformin—a new old drug." Endokrynologia Polska 68, no. 4 (2017): 482–496.
17. Johnston, Atholl, and David W. Holt. "Immunosuppressant drugs–the role of therapeutic drug monitoring." British Journal of Clinical Pharmacology 52, no. Suppl 1 (2001): 61S.
18. Shah, P. M. "The need for new therapeutic agents: What is in the pipeline." Clinical Microbiology and Infection 11 (2005): 36–42.
19. Xue, Xuejia, Feng Wang, and Xiaogang Liu. "Emerging functional nanomaterials for therapeutics." Journal of Materials Chemistry 21, no. 35 (2011): 13107–13127.
20. Patra, Jayanta Kumar, Gitishree Das, Leonardo Fernandes Fraceto, Estefania Vangelie Ramos Campos, Maria del Pilar Rodriguez-Torres, Laura Susana Acosta-Torres, Luis Armando Diaz-Torres et al. "Nano based drug delivery systems: Recent developments and future prospects." Journal of Nanobiotechnology 16, no. 1 (2018): 1–33.
21. Anasori, B., Lukatskaya, M. R., Gogotsi, Y. "2D metal carbides and nitrides (MXenes) for energy storage." Nature Reviews Materials 2, no. 2(2017):16098.
22. Chaturvedi, K., V. Hada, S. Paul, B. Sarma, D. Malvi, M. Dhangar, H. Bajpai, A. Singhwane, A. K. Srivastava, and S. Verma. "The rise of MXene: A wonder 2D material, from its synthesis and properties to its versatile applications—A comprehensive review." Topics in Current Chemistry 381, no. 2(2023):11.
23. Raliya, R., & P. Biswas. "MXene composites for biomedical applications: Current status and future perspectives." Advanced Healthcare Materials 7, no. 23 (2018):1801135.

24. Brown, Joel S., Sarah R. Amend, Robert H. Austin, Robert A. Gatenby, Emma U. Hammarlund, and Kenneth J. Pienta. "Updating the definition of cancer." Molecular Cancer Research 21, no. 11 (2023): 1142–1147.
25. Fitzgerald, Rebecca C., Antonis C. Antoniou, Ljiljana Fruk, and Nitzan Rosenfeld. "The future of early cancer detection." Nature Medicine 28, no. 4 (2022): 666–677.
26. Bhatia, Sangeeta N., Xiaoyuan Chen, Marina A. Dobrovolskaia, and Twan Lammers. "Cancer nanomedicine." Nature Reviews Cancer 22, no. 10 (2022): 550–556.
27. Maleki, Aziz, Matineh Ghomi, Nasser Nikfarjam, Mahsa Akbari, Esmaeel Sharifi, Mohammad-Ali Shahbazi, Mehraneh Kermanian et al. "Biomedical applications of MXene-integrated composites: Regenerative medicine, infection therapy, cancer treatment, and biosensing." Advanced Functional Materials 32, no. 34 (2022): 2203430.
28. Singhwane A, Chaturvedi K, Mohapatra RK, Srivastava AK, Verma S. Mxene-Based Composite Materials as Antibacterial Agents for Healthcare Applications. In Age of MXenes, Volume 2. Applications in Diagnostics, Therapeutics, and Environmental Remediation 2023. American Chemical Society, 2023, pp. 1–17.
29. Lin, Yiyi, Shibo Xu, Xingjun Zhao, Linna Chang, Yanan Hu, Zhenhua Chen, Xifan Mei, and Dong Chen. "Preparation of NIR-sensitive, photothermal and photodynamic multi-functional Mxene nanosheets for laryngeal cancer therapy by regulating mitochondrial apoptosis." Materials & Design 220 (2022): 110887.
30. Vahid Mohammadi, Armin, Johanna Rosen, and Yury Gogotsi. "The world of two-dimensional carbides and nitrides (MXenes)." Science 372, no. 6547 (2021): eabf1581.
31. Tahir, Muhammad. "Vanadium carbide (V2CT x) MXene-supported exfoliated g-C_3N_4 with the role of hole scavenger as a rapid electron transfer channel for enhancing photocatalytic CO_2reduction to CO and CH_4." Energy & Fuels 37, no. 14 (2023): 10615–10630.
32. Hao, Zining, Yifei Li, Xiaoying Liu, Tian Jiang, Yuchu He, Xuwu Zhang, Cong Cong, Desong Wang, Zhiwei Liu, and Dawei Gao. "Enhancing biocatalysis of a MXene-based biomimetic plasmonic assembly for targeted cancer treatments in NIR-II biowindow." Chemical Engineering Journal 425 (2021): 130639.
33. Liu, Yunxiu, Qiuyang Han, Weizhong Yang, Xueqi Gan, Yuanyi Yang, Kenan Xie, Lu Xie, and Yi Deng. "Two-dimensional MXene/cobalt nanowire heterojunction for controlled drug delivery and chemo-photothermal therapy." Materials Science and Engineering: C 116 (2020): 111212.
34. Feng, Xin, Mingjun Li, Jianming Wang, Xianrui Zou, Hongshui Wang, Donghui Wang, Huan Zhou, Lei Yang, Wei Gao, and Chunyong Liang. "MXene quantum dot/zeolitic imidazolate framework nanocarriers for dual stimulus triggered tumor chemo-phototherapy." Materials 15, no. 13 (2022): 4543.
35. Zhang, Xiaoge, Lili Cheng, Yao Lu, Junjie Tang, Qijun Lv, Xiaomei Chen, You Chen, and Jie Liu. "A MXene-based bionic cascaded-enzyme nanoreactor for tumor phototherapy/enzyme dynamic therapy and hypoxia-activated chemotherapy." Nano-Micro Letters 14 (2022): 1–21.

36. Xing, Chenyang, Shiyou Chen, Xin Liang, Quan Liu, Mengmeng Qu, Qingshuang Zou, Jihao Li et al. "Two-dimensional MXene (Ti3C2)-integrated cellulose hydrogels: Toward smart three-dimensional network nanoplatforms exhibiting light-induced swelling and bimodal photothermal/chemotherapy anticancer activity." ACS Applied Materials & Interfaces 10, no. 33 (2018): 27631–27643.
37. Xu, Yunjie, Yingwei Wang, Jusung An, Adam C. Sedgwick, Mingle Li, Jianlei Xie, Weibin Hu, et al. "2D-ultrathin MXene/DOXjade platform for iron chelation chemo-photothermal therapy." Bioactive Materials 14 (2022): 76–85.
38. Hussein, Essraa A., Moustafa M. Zagho, Balsam R. Rizeq, Nadin N. Younes, Gianfranco Pintus, Khaled A. Mahmoud, Gheyath K. Nasrallah, and Ahmed A. Elzatahry. "Plasmonic MXene-based nanocomposites exhibiting photothermal therapeutic effects with lower acute toxicity than pure MXene." International Journal of Nanomedicine 14 (2019): 4529–4539. https://doi.org/10.2147/IJN.S202208
39. Sun, Kuo-Yang, Yizhang Wu, Jia Xu, Wenfang Xiong, Wei Xu, Jiawei Li, Ziying Sun et al. "Niobium carbide (MXene) reduces UHMWPE particle-induced osteolysis." Bioactive Materials 8 (2022): 435–448.
40. Liu, Aiping, Yan Liu, Gengjun Liu, Aitang Zhang, Yujun Cheng, Ying Li, Lin Zhang et al. "Engineering of surface modified $Ti_3C_2T_x$ MXene based dually controlled drug release system for synergistic multitherapies of cancer." Chemical Engineering Journal 448 (2022): 137691.
41. Zada, Shah, Wenhao Dai, Zhang Kai, Huiting Lu, Xiangdan Meng, Yiyi Zhang, Yaru Cheng, et al. "Algae extraction controllable delamination of vanadium carbide nanosheets with enhanced near-infrared photothermal performance." Angewandte Chemie International Edition 59, no. 16 (2020): 6601–6606.

9

MXene-Based Materials for Wound Healing

Manal M. Khan, Gaurav Chaturvedi, Ved Prakash Rao, and Madhuri Arora

9.1 Introduction

The skin is the largest organ in the human body, and can weigh up to 11 kg in people weighing 75 kg or more. Furthermore, the skin encompasses every exterior area of the body. It serves as the body's first line of defense against pathogen infection, the damaging effects of UVA and UVB radiation, physical trauma, heat exchange, and excessive moisture loss [1]. The three layers that comprise this organ are the dermis, epidermis, and hypodermis. Skin tissue must develop and heal from damage throughout a person's lifetime. Wounds are distinguished by ruptured cellular integrity and, depending on their severity, can reveal fascia, blood vessels, and even the area beneath bones. Burns and incisions/excisions brought on by surgery or trauma are the most common types [2,3]. Following an injury, wound healing is an essential biological process that restores tissue integrity and functionality. It includes several painstakingly planned processes involving intricate molecular and cellular interactions. Comprehending the complexities of wound healing is essential for managing acute injuries, but it also has important consequences for wounds that persist, which frequently present considerable clinical difficulties. Dressings in films, hydrogels [4,5], sprays, and composites are applied to the injury site to prevent damage. Conventional dressings for wounds, like bandages, gauze, wool, and cotton have drawbacks such as poor exudate absorption, pathogen penetration, and the need to remove the materials after the lesion heals, which can damage the repaired skin tissue [6]. One development made to address these shortcomings has been the creation of films based on biopolymers for wound healing, which feature thin structure, flexibility, and transparency. Some benefits of these systems include that they can be used as a temporary covering for damaged skin, have mechanical flexibility, control the release of medications, monitor the wound-healing process, and have swelling qualities that collect exudates from the wound bed [7].

DOI: 10.1201/9781003353287-9

Research on wound healing has progressed, resulting in a deeper comprehension of the fundamental mechanisms and the creation of novel therapeutic approaches. This introduction sets the tone for a study into the multidimensional realm of wound healing, trying to solve the secrets of tissue restoration. This dynamic process is the focus of ongoing research and discovery, from the initial hemostasis and inflammatory response to the latter phases of proliferation and remodeling [8,9].

Recent groundbreaking developments in biomaterials technology have driven a revolutionary transformation within the sector of wound repair. The coming together of multidisciplinary research has made innovative methods possible, which have redefined conventional paradigms in wound care [10]. From sophisticated hydrogels to precisely designed scaffolds, biomaterials have become key components in coordinating the complex web of molecular and cellular processes necessary for the best possible wound healing. The subject of customized biomaterials manufacturing has gained a new perspective with the incorporation of 3D printing techniques, which enable exceptional precision and patient-specific customization. In addition to offering structural support, these biomaterials function as reservoirs for growth factors and bioactive substances that actively encourage tissue regeneration. Advanced biomaterials and biological systems working together synergistically have opened up new possibilities for faster healing, less scarring, and better overall patient outcomes.

This chapter covers the recent advances in wound healing, emphasizing the revolutionary effects of hydrogels, scaffolds, 3D printing, and biomaterials. The chapter also explores the vital role of MXenes in the healing process, emphasizing the diverse qualities that render them invaluable in the generation of cutting-edge materials for efficient and expedited wound healing. It also looks at the prospective directions these advances could go in determining the future direction of wound care. The chapter seeks to condense the current state of the art regarding wound healing, setting the stage for a more in-depth examination of recent developments, cutting-edge technologies, and exciting new directions in the quest to improve the healing process for people with various wound challenges.

9.2 Wound Healing: A Complex Journey to Tissue Restoration

Healing a wound is a dynamic and intricate process that the body undergoes to repair damaged tissues and restore their standard structure and function. This multifaceted journey involves various events orchestrated by multiple cells, growth factors, and extracellular matrix components. This chapter delves into the phases of wound healing, the cellular players involved, and the factors influencing this essential biological process [11].

9.2.1 Wound-Healing Phases

Healing a wound is dynamic and multifaceted, with multiple overlapping phases. Wound healing occurs in three basic phases, as shown in Figure 9.1 [12].

9.2.1.1 Inflammatory Phase

Initiated immediately after injury, the inflammatory phase aims to control bleeding, remove debris, and prevent infection. Platelets release clotting factors, and immune cells, such as macrophages and neutrophils, infiltrate the site of the wound to eliminate pathogens and cellular debris.

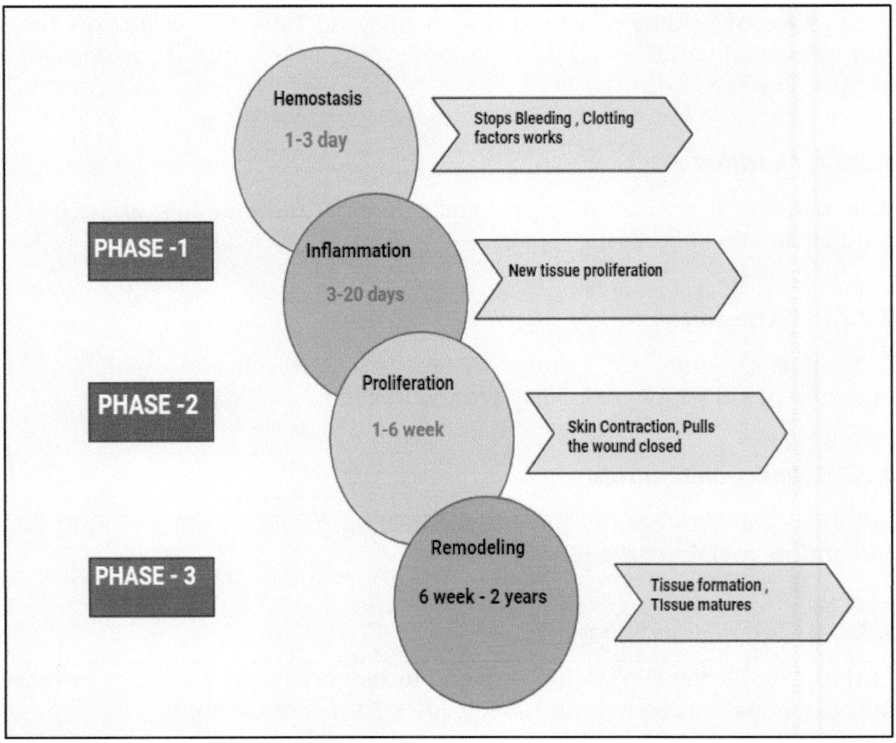

FIGURE 9.1
Flowchart representation of the wound-healing phases.

9.2.1.2 Proliferative Phase

Characterized by the proliferation of new tissue, the proliferative phase involves the fibroblasts' migration and proliferation, synthesis of a new extracellular matrix, and new blood vessel development (angiogenesis). Collagen, a key structural protein, is deposited to strengthen the healing tissue.

9.2.1.3 Remodeling Phase

The maturation or remodeling phase can last for a few months to years. The initially deposited collagen is rearranged and remodeled during this phase to enhance tissue strength. The wound undergoes contraction, and scar tissue formation occurs.

9.2.2 Factors Influencing Wound Healing

In order to repair injured tissues and regain standard structure and function, the process of healing a wound is dynamic and intricate, as it takes time. Some essential variables influencing the healing of wounds are as described in the following [13].

9.2.2.1 Nutrition

Adequate nutrition, including proteins, vitamins, and minerals, is crucial for cellular function and tissue repair.

9.2.2.2 Oxygenation

Oxygen is essential for cellular metabolism and collagen synthesis. An impaired blood supply can delay wound healing.

9.2.2.3 Infection Control

Infections can significantly impede the healing process. Proper wound care and antimicrobial interventions are vital.

9.2.2.4 Chronic Conditions

Chronic conditions, such as diabetes and immunodeficiency, can compromise the normal wound-healing process, leading to chronic wounds.

9.3 Recent Advancements in Wound-Healing Materials and Technology

Researchers have been at the forefront of a revolution in materials science and technology for wound healing, which has changed how therapeutic procedures are approached. The field of biomaterials has gained prominence because of the exceptional capacities of hydrogels, nanoparticles, and bioactive dressings to facilitate targeted and rapid tissue repair. In light of researchers' combined efforts, a new age of improved patient outcomes and life quality will shortly begin, one in which the combination of cutting-edge materials and technology has the potential to rewrite the rules for wound care completely.

The study by Barbaz et al. [14] examined the impact of adding different nanoparticles to multicore microcapsules and how this affected the recovery efficacy based on self-healing polymers in microcapsules. The improved microcapsules by multiwalled carbon nanotubes (MWCNTs), nanoclay, and nanosilica were introduced into the polymers through fabrication. To the epoxy matrix, three-volume fractions of microcapsules at 5%, 7.5%, and 10% were added. To find the healing effectiveness of synthetically produced self-healing polymers, the maximum tensile stresses of the virgin specimens disrupted by a compression impact test and the repaired specimens were measured. In order to anticipate the healing efficiencies, by using the development of representative volume elements (RVEs) and the ABAQUS-Explicit solver linked to VUSDFLD subroutines, a multi-scale finite element (FE) modeling was also encouraged. The results suggested that specimen healing efficiency was increased by raising the volume fractions (VFs) of microcapsules. The likelihood of encountering low-velocity impact (LVI) test-induced cracks with microcapsules may rise with increasing VF of the microcapsules. Therefore, specimens with higher VF of microcapsules would mend more efficiently if healing chemicals were widely disseminated into the propagating cracks. Additionally, the effectiveness of specimen healing was decreased when microcapsule strength was increased. For illustration, the effectiveness of healing was 50.41% for enhanced microcapsules with nanosilica and 45.90% for samples with 10% VF of improved microcapsules using MWCNTs. Enhancing the mechanical characteristics of microcapsules may reduce the likelihood of broken microcapsules, decreasing the specimens' ability to mend. Lastly, the accuracy of the anticipated healing efficiency of the simulated RVEs was better, demonstrating the validity of the multi-scale finite element method (FEM) that was introduced.

Multimodal wearable devices, the basis for 'smart' bandages, may allow for active wound healing and real-time physiological monitoring. Still, there hasn't been much progress in integrating stimulators and sensors into the smart bandage technologies available today. Furthermore, the detachment of sticky dressings without switchable adhesion might cause additional injury to fragile wound tissues, even if adhesive electrodes are necessary for strong signal transmission. Jiang et al. in 2023 [15] addressed these problems by creating a flexible bioelectronic system that consists of hydrogel electrodes that interface with the skin and can attach and disconnect on demand. The circuits in the system are closed-loop, wirelessly powered circuits for stimulation and sensing. They show our wound care system can deliver electrical stimulation in response to the wound environment and continually measure skin impedance and temperature in mice. In comparison to the control group, the treatment group healed around 25% faster and had a 50% improvement in dermal remodeling across preclinical wound types. Additionally, they saw that populations of monocytes and macrophages have activated pro-regenerative genes. This could improve skin healing, neovascularization, and tissue regeneration.

In 2023, Zuo and colleagues [16] designed a biosphere technique to enhance stem cell encapsulation for therapeutic use. The criteria for drug administration, material feasibility, yield, and cell viability are all met by this process. Through a battery of tests, they showed that encapsulated adipose-derived stromal cells (ADSCs) are guaranteed to be bioavailable and functional through the use of biospheres. Additionally, they showed that biosynspheres shield ADSCs from the harshness of clinical handling procedures such as cryopreservation, syringe/nozzle injection, high-speed centrifugation, and thawing. An in vivo investigation using pigs with complete skin defects further demonstrated the superior wound-healing capabilities of this innovative biosynsphere technology. The findings demonstrated that biosynspheres were incorporated into the target tissues and aided in the healing of damaged areas by hastening the process of healing, lowering the production of scar tissue, and returning the ratio of type I to type III collagen deposition to normal. These results highlight the biosynsphere's potential as a better biofabrication technique for tissue regeneration in a medical context. A gentle microfluidic technique is used to encapsulate stem cells in biomaterials that are ready for therapeutic use. With this method, stem cells are guaranteed to remain stable after encapsulation. The produced biosynspheres' production and viability satisfy drug administration regulations. The encapsulated stem cells remained viable and functional, as demonstrated by their capacity to infuse into intended areas and facilitate the healing of damaged tissue after transplantation.

Bio-inks based on oxidized sodium alginate (OSA), sodium alginate, and calcium carbonate microspheres were made for this investigation by Lin and other colleagues in 2023 [17]. To improve printability, Ca^{2+} was pre-cross-linked into each bio-ink. To treat diabetic wounds, porous hydrogel scaffolds were created via 3D printing, as shown in Figure 9.2. $CaCO_3$ was added to the bio-ink to act as a calcium supply and perhaps neutralize the acid in wounds caused by chronic diabetes. Scanning electron microscopy, nuclear

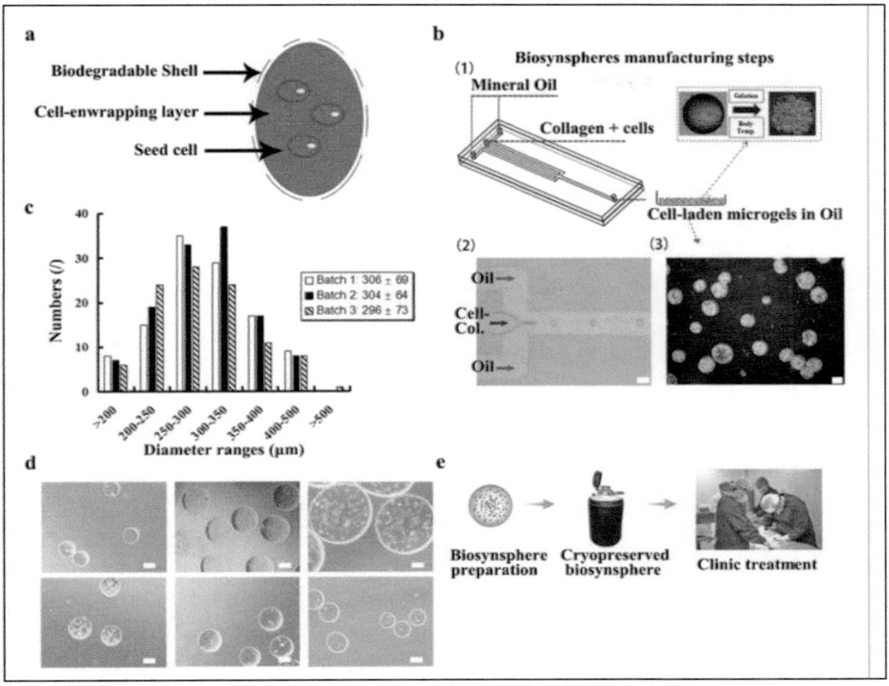

FIGURE 9.2
(a) Systematic representation of the framework of a biosynsphere. (b) Conceptual representation of a biosynsphere construction process (bottom-left scale bar: 500 μm; bottom-right scale bar: 200 μm). (c) The dispersion of biosynsphere sizes throughout three consecutive batches, with a goal average size of 300 μm. (d) Microscopic photographs of biosynspheres with varying diameters and densities of cell (100 μm scale bar). (e) Diagram illustrating the post-fabrication processing of the biosynsphere [16].

magnetic resonance spectroscopy, gel permeation chromatography (GPC), and Fourier-transform infrared spectroscopy (FTIR) were used to characterize these bio-ink components. NIH-3T3 cell proliferation was examined in the samples using the Calcein AM staining and CCK-8 test. In addition, the impact on wound healing was examined by applying the hydrogel scaffolds that are porous to the full-thickness wounds of type I diabetic SD rats (TIDR). When the SA/OSA/gel scaffold was applied to full-thickness wounds on the SD rat back, it expedited wound healing, and increased angiogenesis. It demonstrated 93.0 ± 2.5% collagen deposition between disintegrated hydrogel scaffold fragments. It also merged well with the regenerated tissue. When combined, bio-inks made of OSA, SA, 3Gel, and calcium carbonate can be used to create porous hydrogel scaffolds that can be 3D printed, offering a possible method for enhancing diabetic wound healing (Figure 9.3).

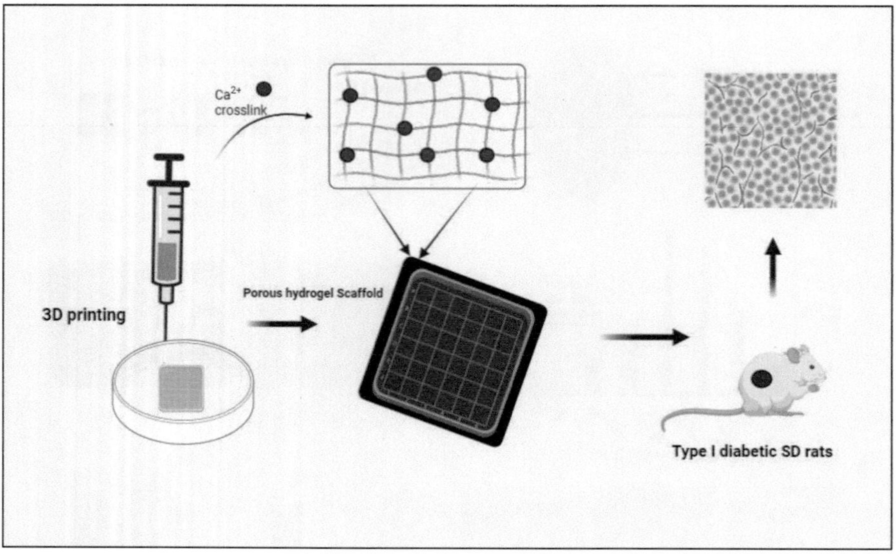

FIGURE 9.3
Framework for the creation of porous hydrogel scaffold by 3D printing technology.

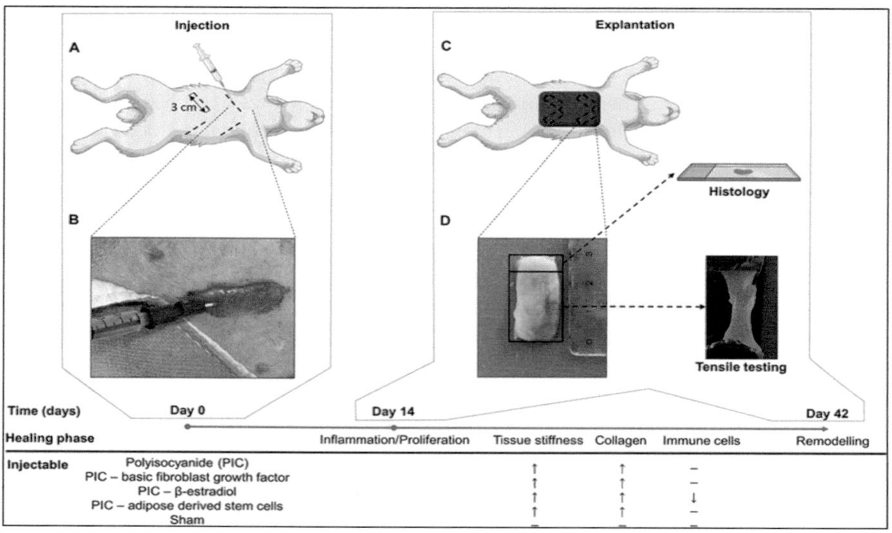

FIGURE 9.4
Surgical technique and explanation. (A) Four hydrogel injection sites and abdominal wall incisions per animal. (B) Injection of hydrogel following cannula closure of the superficial muscle layer. (C, D) Wounds with full thickness (black rectangles) that were excised from the abdomen were prepared for histopathology and tensile testing [18].

In this study, Aksel et al. [18] examined these functionalized gels' application to connective tissue in an in vivo model of an abdominal wound. The objectives are to assess the regeneration capacity of PIC gel in a rabbit's abdominal wound compared to hydrogel-free surgery and to determine which bioactive component enhances healing beyond PIC alone 14 and 42 days after injection. They measured the immune system, connective tissue regeneration, and abdominal wall stiffness to examine healing outcomes connected to the pelvic floor's support role. Applying PIC gel in combination with conjugated bFGF or ADSCs does not adversely impact this healing response; nonetheless, findings point to an E2 moderating effect on PMNC penetration. According to these results and earlier in vivo research, injectable PIC gel can function as a pro-regenerative treatment supplement to treat prolapse repair. Future research is needed to examine the advantageous effects of bFGF and E2, which will be applied to a sheep vaginal wound model that is more translational in nature (Figure 9.4).

9.4 Emerging Technologies in Wound Healing

Advancements in technology continue to drive innovation in wound healing, offering novel approaches to accelerate recovery, reduce complications, and enhance overall patient outcomes. Below are some emerging technologies shaping the landscape of wound healing, as shown in Figure 9.5 [19,20].

9.4.1 Bioprinting and 3D Tissue Engineering

Bioprinting technology allows the accurate cell deposition layer by layer, growth factors, and biomaterials to create three-dimensional tissues. This approach holds promise for fabricating customized skin grafts and complex tissue structures tailored to individual patient needs.

9.4.2 Gene Therapy for Wound Healing

Gene therapy involves the introduction of therapeutic genes into cells to promote specific healing processes. Researchers are exploring gene therapy to enhance growth factor production, angiogenesis, and cell migration in the wound site, ultimately accelerating healing.

9.4.3 Nanotechnology and Nanomedicine

Nanoparticles and nanomaterials are harnessed for targeted drug delivery, antimicrobial applications, and diagnostic purposes. Nanomedicine allows

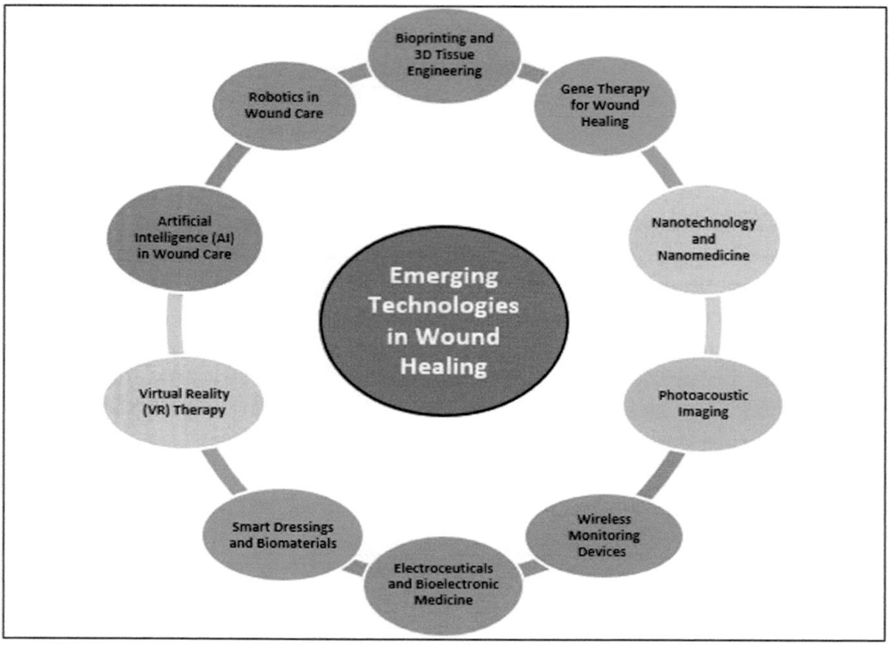

FIGURE 9.5
The emerging technologies in wound healing.

for precise control over therapeutic interventions at the molecular level, offering potential solutions for chronic wounds and infections.

9.4.4 Photoacoustic Imaging

Photoacoustic imaging yields high-resolution images of blood vessels and tissue structures by combining optical and laser-induced ultrasound. This non-invasive imaging technique aids in the real-time monitoring of wound-healing processes, facilitating the early identification of issues.

9.4.5 Wireless Monitoring Devices

Wearable and implantable devices with sensors continuously monitor wound parameters, including temperature, moisture, and pH levels. These wireless devices provide healthcare professionals with real-time data for timely intervention and personalized treatment plans.

9.4.6 Electroceuticals and Bioelectronic Medicine

Bioelectronic devices deliver electrical impulses to modulate neural signals and regulate physiological processes. Electroceuticals show promise in wound healing by influencing inflammation, immune responses, and tissue regeneration. Implantable devices can be targeted to specific nerves related to wound healing.

9.4.7 Artificial Intelligence (AI) in Wound Care

AI algorithms analyze various data sources, including images, patient history, and real-time monitoring data, to provide insights into wound assessment, predict healing trajectories, and optimize treatment strategies. AI-driven tools enhance clinical decision-making and improve patient outcomes.

9.4.8 Smart Dressings and Biomaterials

Smart materials are used in advanced wound dressings, which react to changes in the wound environment. These materials may release therapeutic agents, sense infection, or provide sustained release of growth factors. Biomimetic materials mimic the natural extracellular matrix, promoting cell attachment and tissue regeneration.

9.4.9 Virtual Reality (VR) Therapy

VR is being explored as a therapeutic tool to manage pain and improve patient outcomes during wound care. Immersive VR environments can distract patients, reduce anxiety, and enhance their overall experience, potentially facilitating faster healing.

9.4.10 Robotics in Wound Care

Robotic systems are being developed to assist in wound debridement, a critical process in removing dead tissue. Robotics can enhance precision and reduce the risk of infection by automating certain aspects of wound care procedures [21].

These emerging technologies represent a transformative era in wound healing, offering a diverse range of approaches to address the complexities of tissue repair. As research and development in these areas continue, integrating these technologies into clinical practice can revolutionize the standard of care for patients with acute and chronic wounds

9.5 MXene's Breakthrough Role in Advancing Wound Healing

Recently, MXene materials have attracted a lot of interest because of their revolutionary contribution to the advancement of wound healing. MXenes exhibit unmatched potential in expediting and facilitating successful wound repair due to their distinct blend of superior electrical conductivity, biological compatibility, and mechanical strength. Additionally, MXenes have natural antibacterial qualities that reduce the chance of infections at wound sites. Recent advancements in the comprehension of and ability to harness MXenes' diverse properties indicate a bright future for the development of novel materials that possess the capacity to completely transform the field of wound healing.

T-RMFs containing vitamin E with controlled release ability for wound healing were developed by Jin et al. in 2021 [22]. These T-RMFs were made out of a thermosensitive PAAV-coating layer and MXene nanosheets dispersed over composite nanobelts made of polyacrylonitrile and polyvinylpyrrolidone, as shown in Figure 9.6. The MXene nanosheets' large surface area and high mass loading give the T-RMFs exceptional photothermal capabilities. By exposing the material to near-infrared (NIR) irradiation, the temperature could be readily adjusted. Subsequently, the interface was loosened by the thermoresponsive polymeric coating layer, allowing vitamin E to dissolve and encouraging its release. In cellular and animal experiments, the T-RMFs showed outstanding wound-healing and biocompatibility capabilities. The

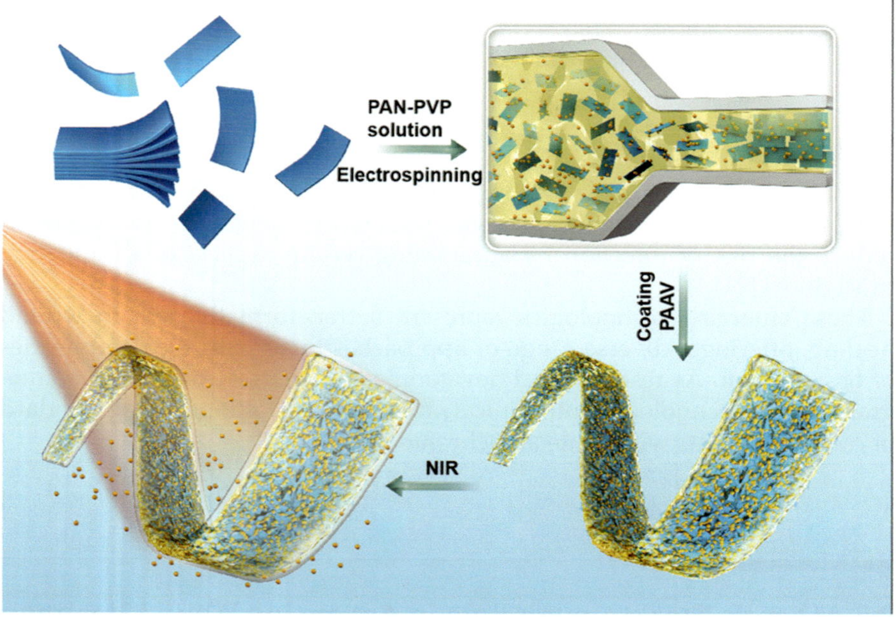

FIGURE 9.6
Design for the surface coating and fabrication of T-RMF nanobelts [23].

excellent wound-healing functions, high surface area, mass production potential, interesting nanobelt/nanosheets structure, easy method, and NIR responsive properties of these T-RMFs suggest that our nanobelts have great possible outcomes for tissue engineering, wound healing, and much broader application areas. This easy way to make nanobelts and nanosheets creates new opportunities for the production and use of nanomaterials.

In their study, Li and colleagues in 2022 [23] provided a straightforward method for creating an antimicrobial, healable, and injectable MXene hydrogel. This was achieved by incorporating the antibacterial MXene nanosheets coated with silver nanoparticles structure into a guar gum and phenylboronic acid-fused sodium alginate (Alg-PBA) polymer network. This allows for portable human–machine interaction and exceptional human healthcare monitoring, including potential rehabilitation training, the diagnosis of heart and muscle diseases, and efficient wound therapy with significantly accelerated wound healing. The as-prepared MXene hydrogel (AgNPs/MXene/GG/Alg-PBA) showed improved electrical conductivity, stronger mechanical strength, and strong antibacterial activity as a result of the addition of antibacterial AgNPs/MXene nanosheets. The multipurpose epidermic sensors known as MXene hydrogel were designed to monitor both large human activities and small electrophysiological signals, such as ECG and EMG, with great sensitivity. This allows the hydrogel to provide crucial clinical data for the treatment of disorders connected to the heart and muscles, as well as rehabilitation training. The MXene hydrogel has remarkable self-healing properties because of the supramolecular interactions between silver NPs/MXene nanosheets, guar gum, and Alg-PBA, in addition to the dynamic cross-linking between GG's hydroxyl groups and Alg-PBA's phenyl boronic acid groups. Additionally, as-prepared MXene hydrogel—which is mostly produced from silver NPs coated on MXene nanosheets—showed exceptional antibacterial capabilities in in vitro experiments. The MXene hydrogel's strong injectability, strong self-healing ability, and consistent antibacterial characteristic allowed it to be injected directly into the wound site for additional antibacterial and healing benefits.

In order to promote wound healing, Sun et al. [24] provided new MXene-integrated microneedle patches containing adenosine encapsulation in their study. As seen in Figure 9.7(a), the intended microneedle patches for the experiment were developed using a template replication technique. The 3-(acrylamido)phenylboronic acid- (PBA-)integrated polyethylene glycol diacrylate (PEGDA) hydrogel was utilized as the microneedle patch's host material because of the boronate molecules' dynamic ability to form covalent bonds with adenosine. Because of MXene's ability to convert photothermally, the release of loaded adenosine may be amplified under NIR irradiation to maintain the activation signal close to the injury site. The capability of adenosine-encapsulated MXene-integrated microneedle patches to stimulate angiogenesis was demonstrated by in vitro cell tests. It was shown that the

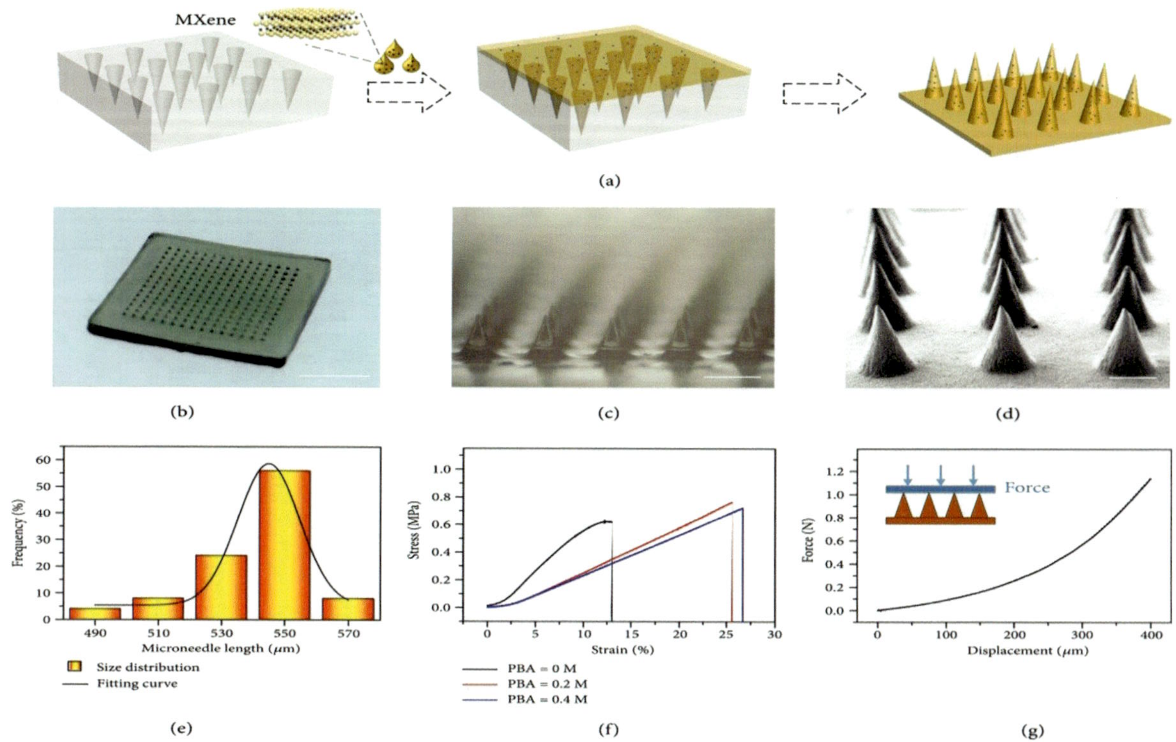

FIGURE 9.7
(A) Schematic illustration showing how microneedle patches are developed. (b) An optical picture of the hydrogel microneedle patch integrated with MXene. (c) A microscopy image enlarging the microneedle array's morphology. (d) A picture of the microneedle patch taken using a scanning electron microscope (SEM). (e) Statistics on the microneedle array's uniformity. (f) The hydrogel patch's stress–strain curves at various PBA concentrations. (g) Testing the microneedle patch's compressive force. The scale bars in (b), (c), and (d) are 4 mm, 400 μm, and 200 μm, respectively [24].

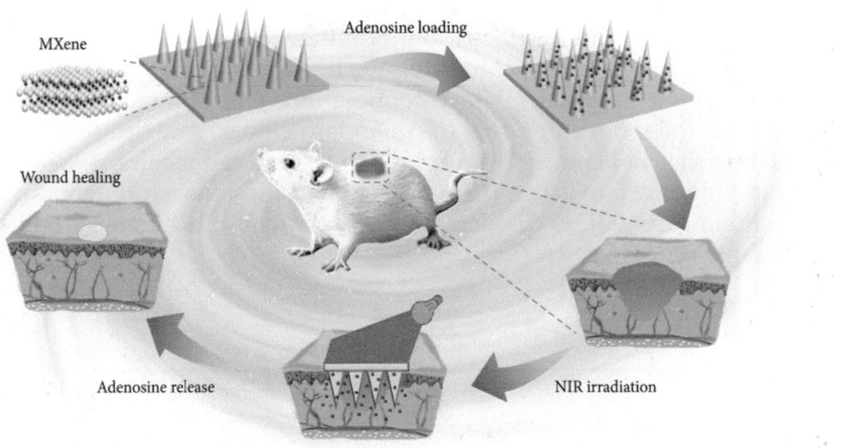

FIGURE 9.8
Demonstrating the way adenosine encapsulation in MXene-integrated microneedle patches promotes wound healing [24].

microneedle patches effectively stimulate angiogenesis, which is conducive to wound healing, as shown in Figure 9.8, when used to treat animal models. Due to these characteristics, the suggested microneedle patch has the potential to be used in wound healing.

9.6 Conclusion and Future Perspectives

Researchers have been at the forefront of a revolution in materials science and technology for wound healing, which has changed how therapeutic procedures are approached. The field of biomaterials has gained prominence because of the exceptional capacities of hydrogels, nanoparticles, and bioactive dressings to facilitate targeted and rapid tissue repair. In light of these researchers' combined efforts, a new age of improved patient outcomes and life quality will shortly begin, one in which the combination of cutting-edge materials and technology has the potential to rewrite the rules for wound care completely. In the future, more investigation and clinical applications will be necessary to enhance these technologies, resolve outstanding issues, and guarantee broad accessibility. The subject of wound healing could undergo a revolution attributable to the novel materials that could be developed, as demonstrated by the recent advancements in comprehending and utilizing MXenes' diverse properties. Future perspectives in wound-healing research should focus on refining and expanding the use of sophisticated biomaterials, enhancing the integration of digital technologies, and developing multidisciplinary cooperation. The ultimate objective is to incorporate these developments into standard clinical practice so that people navigating the challenges of wound rehabilitation can receive more effective and individualized treatment. The direction of these developments suggests that wound care will be characterized by accuracy, effectiveness, and better patient outcomes in the future.

References

1. Saraiva, M.M., Campelo, M.D.S., Camara Neto, J.F., Lima, A.B.N., Silva, G.D.A., Dias, A.T.D.F.F., Ricardo, N.M.P.S., Kaplan, D.L. and Ribeiro, M.E.N.P., 2023. Alginate/polyvinyl alcohol films for wound healing: Advantages and challenges. Journal of Biomedical Materials Research Part B: Applied Biomaterials, 111(1), pp. 220–233.
2. Torkaman S, Rahmani H, Ashori A, Najafi SHM., 2021. Modification of chitosan using amino acids for wound healing purposes: A review. Carbohydrate Polymers, 258, p. 117675. Doi:10.1016/j.carbpol.2021.117675.
3. Pissarenko, A. and Meyers, M.A., 2021. Reprint of the materials science of skin: Analysis, characterization, and modeling. Progress in Materials Science, 120, p. 100816. https://doi.org/10.1016/j.pmatsci.2021.100816
4. Mahmood, H., Khan, I.U., Asif, M., et al., 2021. In vitro and in vivo evaluation of gellan gum hydrogel films: Assessing the co impact of therapeutic oils and ofloxacin on wound healing. International Journal of Biological Macromolecules, 166, pp. 483–495. https://doi.org/10.1016/j.ijbiomac.2020.10.206
5. Zheng, G., Zhang, D., Tang, Q., Ma, H. and Dong, X., 2021. Charge-switchable, anti-oxidative molecule tuned polyelectrolyte multilayered films: Amplified polyelectrolyte diffusivity and accelerated diabetes wound healing. Chemical Engineering Journal, 416, p. 129521. https://doi.org/10.1016/j.cej.2021.129521
6. Okur, M.E., Karantas, I.D., Şenyiğit, Z., Üstündağ Okur, N. and Siafaka, P.I., 2020. Recent trends on wound management: New therapeutic choices based on polymeric carriers. Asian Journal of Pharmaceutical Sciences, 15, pp. 661–684. https://doi.org/10.1016/j.ajps.2019.11.008
7. Moeini, A., Pedram, P., Makvandi, P., Malinconico, M. and d'Ayala, G.G., 2020. Wound healing and antimicrobial effect of active secondary metabolites in chitosan-based wound dressings: A review. Carbohydrate Polymers, 233, p. 115839. https://doi.org/10.1016/j.carbpol.2020.115839
8. Guo, S.A. and DiPietro, L.A., 2010. Factors affecting wound healing. Journal of Dental Research, 89(3), pp. 219–229.

9. Gonzalez, A.C.D.O., Costa, T.F., Andrade, Z.D.A. and Medrado, A.R.A.P., 2016. Wound healing—A literature review. Anais brasileiros de dermatologia, 91, pp. 614–620.
10. Las Heras, K., Igartua, M., Santos-Vizcaino, E. and Hernandez, R.M., 2020. Chronic wounds: Current status, available strategies and emerging therapeutic solutions. Journal of Controlled Release, 328, pp. 532–550. https://doi.org/10.1016/j.jconrel.2020.09.039
11. Witte, M.B. and Barbul, A., 1997. General principles of wound healing. Surgical Clinics of North America, 77(3), pp. 509–528.
12. Schreml, S., Szeimies, R.M., Prantl, L., Landthaler, M. and Babilas, P., 2010. Wound healing in the 21st century. Journal of the American Academy of Dermatology, 63(5), pp. 866–881.
13. Guo, S.A. and DiPietro, L.A., 2010. Factors affecting wound healing. Journal of Dental Research, 89(3), pp. 219–229.
14. Barbaz-Isfahani, R., Saber-Samandari, S. and Salehi, M., 2023. Experimental and numerical research on healing performance of reinforced microcapsule-based self-healing polymers using nanoparticles. Journal of Reinforced Plastics and Composites, 42(3–4), pp. 95–109. https://doi.org/10.1177/07316844221102945
15. Jiang, Y., Trotsyuk, A.A., Niu, S., et al., 2023. Wireless, closed-loop, smart bandage with integrated sensors and stimulators for advanced wound care and accelerated healing. Nature Biotechnology, 41, pp. 652–662. https://doi.org/10.1038/s41587-022-01528-3
16. Lin, Z., Xie, W., Cui, Z., Huang, J., Cao, H. and Li, Y., 2023. 3D printed alginate/gelatin-based porous hydrogel scaffolds to improve diabetic wound healing. Giant, 16, 100185, ISSN2666-5425. https://doi.org/10.1016/j.giant.2023.100185.
17. Zuo, X., Jiang, X., Zhang, Y., Huang Y., Wang, N., Zhu P. and James Kang, Y., 2023. A clinical feasible stem cell encapsulation ensures an improved wound healing. Biomedical Materials, 18(2), p. 025005. https://doi.org/10.1088/1748-605X/acb67a
18. Gudde, A.N., van Velthoven, M.J.J., Kouwer, P.H.J., Roovers, J.-P.W.R. and Guler, Z., 2023. Injectable polyisocyanide hydrogel as healing supplement for connective tissue regeneration in an abdominal wound model. Biomaterials, 302, p. 122337, ISSN 0142-9612. https://doi.org/10.1016/j.biomaterials.2023.122337
19. Chouhan, D., Dey, N., Bhardwaj, N. and Mandal, B.B., 2019. Emerging and innovative approaches for wound healing and skin regeneration: Current status and advances. Biomaterials, 216, p. 119267.
20. Shrestha, B., DeLuna, F., Anastasio, M.A., Yong Ye, J. and Brey, E.M., 2020. Photoacoustic imaging in tissue engineering and regenerative medicine. Tissue Engineering Part B: Reviews, 26(1), pp. 79–102.
21. Guntur, S.R., Gorrepati, R.R. and Dirisala, V.R., 2019. Robotics in healthcare: An internet of medical robotic things (IoMRT) perspective. In Machine learning in bio-signal analysis and diagnostic imaging (pp. 293–318). Academic Press.
22. Jin, L., Guo, X., Gao, D., et al., 2021. NIR-responsive MXene nanobelts for wound healing. NPG Asia Materials, 13, p. 24. https://doi.org/10.1038/s41427-021-00289-w

23. Li, M., Zhang, Y., Lian, L., Liu, K., Lu, M., Chen, Y., Zhang, L., Zhang, X. and Wan, P., 2022. Flexible accelerated-wound-healing antibacterial MXene-based epidermic sensor for intelligent wearable human-machine interaction. Advanced Functional Materials, 32(47), p. 2208141.
24. Sun, L., Fan, L., Bian, F., Chen, G., Wang, Y. and Zhao, Y., 2021. MXene-integrated microneedle patches with innate molecule encapsulation for wound healing. Research, 2021. DOI: 10.34133/2021/9838490.

Index

A

ABAQUS, 141
Accordion, 26–27
Acetaminophen (ACOP), 35
Acetylcholinesterase, 19
ACHMS scaffold, 73
Adaptability, 90
Adenocarcinomas, 39
Adhesive patches, 90
Adipose-derived stromal cells (ADSCs), 142
AF fibroblasts, 73
Aflatoxin B1 (AFB1), 22
Alkaline phosphatase, 115
American Cancer Society, 36
Amino silane, 25
Anesthetics, 121
Anti-carcinoembryonic antigen antibodies (Ab1), 25
Antibacterial, 53
Antibacterial/antimicrobial properties, 12
Antibiotics, 121
Antibody, 21
Anticancer agents, 121
Anticancer treatment, 128
Antidepressants, 121
Antifouling behavior, 19
Anti-inflammatory agents, 121
Antioxidant and anti-inflammatory agents, 128
Antiseptic, 22
Antitumor agents, 121, 124, 128
Antiviral agents, 121
Aortic valve, 92
Arterial palpation, 92
Arterial pulse, 92
Artificial Intelligence (AI) in Wound Care, 147
Athlete performance optimization, 90
Atrial fibrillation, 122
Au@CQDs-MXene, 23
AuNPs/$Ti_3C_2T_x$-PDDA, 23

B

Bandgap, 88
β-hydroxybutyrate dehydrogenase 34
β-hydroxybutyric acid 34
Binding with biomolecules, 55
Bio-inks, 142
Bioanalytical bionsensing, 21
Biochemical analytes in blood serum, 43
Biocompatibility, 7, 19
Biodegradable electronics, 86
Biohybrid platforms, 115
Bioimaging/diagnostic imaging, 10
Biomarkers, 10
Biomedicine, 1
Bioprinting and 3D tissue engineering, 145
Biopsy, 36
Bioreactors, 72
Biosensing, 9
Biosensors, 31
Bladder cancers, 122
Blade coating, 91
Bleaching agent, 22
Blinking rate, 96
Blood biomarkers, 41
Blood clots, 122
Blood glucose, 24
Blood glucose concentration, 37
Blood pressure, 31
Bone repair, 71
Bone-tumor xenografts, 77
Brain-machine interfaces, 127
Breast cancer, 25, 39, 131
Breathing variations 96
Bronchi, 38
Bronchioles, 38
Bronchogenic carcinoma/cancer, 38

C

Calcium carbonate, 142, 143
Cancer antigen-125 (CA125), 40
Cancer antigens, 37

Cancer biomarker, 25
Cancer screening, 18
Carbon fiber membrane (CFM), 98
Carcinoembryonic antigen (CEA), 25
Carcinogenic, 23
Cardiomyocytes, 114
Cartilage restoration, 71
Causing oxidative damage, 55
CEA detection monitor, 25
Cell biology, 71
Cells, 72
Cell seeding, 71
Cell spreading, 115
Cervical cancer mortality, 36
Chemical etching, 52
Chemical sensors, 97
Chemotherapy, 124
Cholesterol level, 31
Chromatography, 35
Chronic conditions, 140
Circulating tumor DNA (ctDNA), 37
Clay matrix, 93
Clinical diagnosis, 86
Clustered Regularly Interspaced Short Palindromic Repeats-12a (CRISPR-12a), 19
CNTs, 94
CNTs/Ti_3C_2/PB electrode, 98
Collagen type I, 115
Colloidal solution, 89
Colorectal, 25
Colorectal cancer, 40
Combination therapies, 127
Corrosion resistance, 111
Creatinine, 42
Crinkled/crumpled morphologies, 20
Cryopreservation, 142
CT, 36
Cytokines, 37
Cytology, 36
Cytotoxic singlet oxygen, 59, 60

D

Degree of dissemination, 38
Dental procedures, 111
Destabilization of membranes, 55
Detecting oncogenesis, 36
Diabetes, 24
Diabetic nephropathy, 41
Diastole, 92
Diastolic component, 92, 93
Dichotic peak, 92
Dip coating, 91
Disease diagnosis, 2
DNA aptamer, 19
Double-stranded 3D DNA walker technology, 19
Doxorubicin, 128
Drug delivery, 127
Drugs, 127

E

E. coli 59
Ecoflex substrate, 97
Elastic stiffness, 109
Elastomers, 90
Electrical conductivity, 1, 2, 6–7, 11, 18–21, 23, 24, 27, 56, 62, 63, 87–90, 94, 95, 98, 103, 115, 123, 126–127, 148, 149
Electroceuticals and bioelectronic medicine, 146
Electrochemical (EC) signaling process, 21
Electrochemical carcinoembryonic antigen biosensor, 25
Electrochemical sensors, 97
Electrochemiluminescence, 26
Electro-chemo-luminescent (ECL), 19
Electrode-electrolyte interface, 98
Electrodes as biomarkers, 35
Electromagnetic interference (EMI) effect, 56
Electromagnetic waves, 56
Electromyography (EMG), 86, 94
Electron-hole pairs in semiconductors, 55
Electron-phonon coupling, 55
Electrospinning, 91
Endogenous, 22
Endoscopy, 36
Enzyme, 21
Enzyme adsorption efficiency, 24
Enzyme biosensors, 21
Enzyme-linked immunosorbent test (ELISA), 36
Enzyme motion, 19
EpCAM antigen, 26
Epigastric pain, 39

Epithelial cell, 40
Epithelium, 40
Erythrocytes, 20
Esophageal cancer, 23
Estrogen receptors, 39
European Group of Tumor Markers (EGTM), 39
Exogenous, 22
Exonuclease III, 26
Exosomes, 37
Eyelid, 96

F

Fabrication Process of the MXene Sensing Layer, 90
Facial expression, 87, 95, 96
Factors Influencing Wound Healing, 140
Fall detection, 90
Fall prevention, 90
Fast Response Time, 90
Fatty liver, 42
Fermi level, 88
Fingerprick test strips, 87
Fitness tracking, 87
Flexible electronics, 86
Flocculation, 20
Flow cytometry, 36
Fluorescence, 22
Fluoride-free, 19
Forster resonance energy transfer (FRET) biosensor, 18
Freeze-drying technique, 93
Functionalized gels, 145

G

Gait analysis, 90
Gas sensors, 100
Gene therapy for wound healing, 145
Genomic and proteomic, 36
Geriatric, 34
Glass carbon electrode (GCE), 23
Glomerular filtration rate, 41
Glucose monitoring, 25
Glucose oxidase (GOx), 24, 130
Glucose sensor, 24
Gold nanoparticle, 18
Gout, 42
GOx loadings, 24
Granulation tissue, 51
Graphite, 89
Growth factors, 72
Gynecological cancer, 40

H

Hb immobilizer 22
HBV-DNA, 26
Heart contracts, 92
Heart rate, 86
Heart tissue engineering, 114
Heart valve scaffold, 74
Helicobacter pylori, 26–27
Hemoglobin, 23
Homophobic, 34
High-speed centrifugation, 142
High surface area and excellent electrical conductivity, 7
HIL microreactor, 22
HIV, 121
HOMO (highest occupied molecular orbital), 55
Human activity monitoring, 94
Human Kallikrein-3 PSA, 43
Human–machine interfaces, 96
Human muscle movements, 94
Hydrogen bonding, 93
Hydrogen peroxide (H_2O_2) sensor, 22
Hydrophilicity, 89
Hydrophobic ionic liquid (HIL), 22
Hydroxyl functionalization, 88
Hyperthermia, 51
Hyperuricemia, 42

I

Imaging, 127
Immune rejection, 70
Immunoassay, 35
Immunohistochemistry (IHC), 36
Immunosensor, 100
Immunotherapy, 124
Implanted gadgets, 86
In situ synthesis, 53
Infection control, 140
Inflammatory phase, 139
Influenza, 121

Inkjet printing, 91
Intercalating agents, 90
Intercalation and delamination, 52, 61
Intervertebral disc regeneration, 74
Isoniazid (INZ), 35

K

Kedambaimoole, 96
Kidney malignancy, 41
Kinetic energy, 54
Kretschmann configuration, 22
Kunming mice, 129

L

Label-free multiplex RNA exploration design, 18
Layer-by-layer assembly, 91
Li+ cations, 88
Liver cancer, 36
Long-term stability, 90
Lower strain regimens, 95
LSPR effect, 56
LUMO (lowest unoccupied molecular orbital), 55
Lung, 25
Lung cancer, 38
Lung malignancy, 38

M

Malignancies, 39
Mass spectrometry, 35
MAX phases, 1, 31, 52, 87, 123, 125
Mechanical flexibility, 1, 2, 7, 11, 90, 103, 136
Mechanical strength, 90
Median sensitivity, 39
Median specificity, 39
Mellitus, 24
Mesothelial cell, 40
Metalloproteinases, 37
Methemoglobinemia, 23
Microcontact printing, 91
Microfluidic station, 22
microRNA, 37
microRNA-155, 26
Migrating cancer cells, 36
MMPs, 37
Moldable/flexible fibers, 101
Monoclonal anti-CEA antibody, 25
MoS_2, 89
Motion and gesture sensing, 96
MQDs (metal-quantum dots), 57
MRI, 36, 127, 129
Mullerian type CA125, 40
multicore microcapsules, 141
multimodal therapy, 60
MWCNTs, 25
MXene-based DNA/aptamer biosensor, 26
MXene-CPAM nanocomposite, 101
MXene/DNA/Pd/Pt, 35
MXene/graphene hybrid fibers, 101
MXene/graphene/AuNPs (MGA), 25
MXene/Pt/C/GCE, 19
MXene/RGO aerogel, 93

N

Nafion/Hb/MXene-Ti_3C_2/GCE, 23
Nafion solution, 35
Nano-perforation, 55
Nanobiotechnology, 50
Nanocapsule, 23
Nano-enzyme, 22
Nanosheets, 19
Nanotechnology and nanomedicine, 145
Nasopharyngeal swabs, 19
National Institutes of Health, 31
Nb_2CT_x MXene, 18
Nb_2CT_x nanosheets, 19
Near-infrared radiation (NIR), 54
Neonatal rat cardiomyocytes (nrCMs), 116
Neural interfaces, 127
Neurotransmitters, 121
NIH-3T3 cell proliferation, 143
NIR laser irradiation, 129
Nitrile sensor, 23
Nitrogenous compounds, 42
Nitrosamines, 23
$NiWO_4$, 20
Nonprotein nitrogen, 42
Nutrition, 140

O

Oncogenic tumors, 36
OncomiRs (microRNA-21 and microRNA-141), 18

Oral squamous cell carcinoma (OSCC), 80
Organ transplantation, 71
Organ transplantation, 73
Organic intercalation, 88
Oscillations, 55
Osteosarcoma, 80
Ovarian, 25
Ovarian cancer, 40
Oxidizing agent, 22
Oxygenation, 140

P

Palliate, 121
Pancreatic, 25
Pancreatic cancer, 39
Peanuts, 22
PEDOT:PSS/MXene/GOx/hydrogel, 24
PEI-Ru@Ti_3C_2@AuNPs, 19
Peptide nucleic acid (PNA), 26
Peroxidase, 22
Perspiration, 98
PHA scaffold, 74
Phosphorene, 108
Photo-induced antimicrobial effects, 55
Photoacoustic imaging, 146
Photodynamic therapy, 50
Photoenergy conversion, 54
Photosensitizers, 60
Photothermal antimicrobial mechanism, 55
Photothermal conversion efficiency (PCE or η), 54, 57, 61, 63, 130, 132
Photothermal conversion mechanism, 56
Photothermal therapy, 10, 50–53, 58, 63, 115, 124, 127–131
Photothermal treatment, 117
Physical therapy sessions, 90
Piezoresistive, 89
Piezoresistive sensor, 89
PLLA-PHA nanofibers, 116
Pluripotent stem cell, 114
Point of care (POC), 18
Poly-L-lysine (PLL), 24
Poly(3,4-ethylene-dioxythiophene), 24
Poly(dimethyl diallyl ammonium chloride), 23
Poly(styrene sulfonate) (PEDOT:PSS), 24
Polyacrylonitrile, 148
Polydopamine, 25, 61
Polymerase chain reaction (PCR), 36
Positron annihilation experiments, 78
Positron emission tomography (PET), 36
Posture monitoring, 90
Potentiostatic deposition technique, 23
Preeclampsia, 41
Pressure sensors, 90
Pressure ulcer prevention, 90
Progesterone receptors, 39
Proliferative phase, 140
Prostate cancer, 43
Prostate inflammation, 43
Prostatic hyperplasia (BPH), 43
Prussian blue, 98
p-type sensing, 101
Pulse monitoring, 92
Pulse waveform, 92
PVA, 93

Q

Quenching, 22
Quercetin, 80, 81

R

Radiation therapy, 124
Radioimmunoassay (RIA), 36
Reactive oxygen species, 22
Real-time reverse transcription amplification (RT-RAA) assay, 19
Regenerative medicine, 2, 3, 5, 7, 9, 12, 13, 14, 70, 71, 73, 81, 113, 127
Rehabilitation exercises, 90
Relaxation of the heart, 92
Remodeling, 137
Remodeling phase, 140
Renal disease, 41
Renal function, 41
Renal impairments, 41
Resonance, 78
Respiration rate, 86
RNA polymerase (RdRp) gene, 19
Robotics in wound care, 147

S

S. aureus, 59, 61
SARS-CoV-2, 18

Scaffolds, 72
Schottky barrier (SB), 101
Screen-printed carbon electrodes (SPCEs), 24
Screen printing, 91
Selective etching method, 3
Self-healing polymers, 141
Semimetal, 56
Sensing layer, 100
Serpentine tunnels, 100
Serum, 19
Signal transmission, 88
Singlet oxygen, 60
6-carboxyfluorescein (FAM), 22
Skin patch, 24
Skin regeneration, 71
Skin temperature, 86
Skin tissue, 137
Smart dressings and biomaterials, 147
Smart textiles, 90
Soft wearable sensors, 86
Sonography, 36
Spiking technique, 20
Spin coating, 91
Spin–orbit coupling, 20
Sports performance tracking, 90
Stamping 91
Staphylococcal, 25
Strain sensor, 93
Substrate, 21
Surface chemical tenability, 1
Surface etched biosensors, 18
Surface functionalization, 53
Surface plasmon resonance (SPR), 22, 25
Surface plasmons, 22
Sweat absorption, 100
Sweat analysis, 98, 101
Sweating, 86
Synthesis methods, 3
Syringe/nozzle injection, 142
Systole 92
Systolic component, 92

T

Tamoxifen, 122
Target analyte, 21
Teratogenic, 23
Tetrapropylammonium hydroxide, 114
Thawing, 142
Therapeutic agents, 3, 9, 11, 121
Therapeutic applications, 53
Thermography, 36
3D bioprinting, 71
3D hybrid sponge, 97
Ti_3C_2-Ag NW-PDA/Ni+ gel, 93
Ti_3C_2-PLL-GOx/GCE, 24
$Ti_3C_2T_x$-PDDA, 23
$Ti_3C_2T_x$-PDDA/GCE, 23
Tidal waves, 92
Tissue, 70
Tissue-engineered vasculature graft (TEVG), 76
Tissue engineering, 10, 71
Tissue regeneration, 11, 112
Tobacco, 124
Tracking and monitoring, 88
Transcriptome, 36
Transdermal glucose monitors, 86
Transducer materials, 98
Transition metal dichalcogenides, 32
Transplant tourism, 70
Transporters, 71
Tricarboxylic acid, 114
Triplet oxygen, 59
Tumor-associated antigens, 41
Tumor formation, 36
Tumor markers, 41
Tumor metastasis, 36
Tunable surface chemistry, 8
2D materials, 1

U

Urate oxidase enzyme, 22
Uric acid, 42
UVA and UVB radiation, 137

V

Valence states, 20
Virtual reality (VR) therapy, 147
Vitamin E, 148
Vocal cord motions, 95
Voice recognition, 87, 95, 96

Volatile organic compounds (VOCs), 101
Voltage, 78

W

Warfarin, 122
Wear and tear, 88
Wearable device applications, 11, 87, 103
Wireless monitoring devices, 146
Wireless sensing technologies, 86
World Health Organization (WHO), 25
Wound healing, 6, 12, 13, 127, 137–152

X

X-ray, 36, 80

Z

Zeolitic imidazolate framework-8 (ZIF-8)
129

For Product Safety Concerns and Information please contact our EU representative GPSR@taylorandfrancis.com Taylor & Francis Verlag GmbH, Kaufingerstraße 24, 80331 München, Germany